IS CROHN'S DISEASE A MYCOBACTERIAL DISEASE?

Developments in Gastroenterology

VOLUME 14

The titles published in this series are listed at the end of this volume.

IS CROHN'S DISEASE A MYCOBACTERIAL DISEASE?

edited by

CHRIS J. J. MULDER
Department of Hepato-gastroenterology,
Rijnstate Hospital,
Arnhem,
The Netherlands

and

GUIDO N. J. TYTGAT
Department of Hepato-gastroenterology,
Academic Medical Centre,
Amsterdam,
The Netherlands

SPRINGER-SCIENCE+BUSINESS MEDIA, B.V.

Library of Congress Cataloging-in-Publication Data

Is Crohn's disease a mycobacterial disease? / edited by Chris J.J.
Mulder and Guido N.J. Tytgat.
p. cm. -- (Developments in gastroenterology ; v. 14)
ISBN 978-94-010-4808-8 ISBN 978-94-011-1830-9 (eBooK)
DOI 10.1007/978-94-011-1830-9
1. Enteritis, Regional--Etiology. 2. Mycobacterial diseases.
I. Mulder, C. J. J. (Chris J. J.) II. Tytgat, G. N. J.
III. Series: Developments in gastroenterology ; 14.
[DNLM: 1. Crohn Disease--etiology. 2. Crohn Disease-
-microbiology. 3. Mycobacterium--pathogenicity. W1 DE997VYB v. 14
/ WI 512 I73]
RC862.E52I8 1993
616.2'445--dc20
DNLM/DLC
for Library of Congress 92-48696

ISBN 978-94-010-4808-8

Printed on acid-free paper

TABLE OF CONTENTS

Introduction

IS CROHN'S DISEASE A MYCOBACTERIAL DISEASE?

The fact that the differential diagnosis of inflammatory bowel disease includes intestinal infections has been a source of much interest and clinical concern for many years. Since the recognition of ulcerative colitis and Crohn's disease as clinical entities, numerous attempts have been made to identify a specific organism resulting in the clinical and pathologic picture of Inflammatory Bowel Disease.

The first suggestion about a connection between Johne's disease, a chronic mycobacterial enteritis in cattle, and Crohn's disease occurred in 1913, when Dalziel described enteritis in humans which, although resembling intestinal tuberculosis, he believed to be a new disorder. Since the work of Crohn in the thirties a few investigators attempted to look for mycobacteria in Crohn's disease.

Until now the work of Van Patter, Burnham and others did not receive widespread recognition. In 1984 the isolation of M. paratuberculosis was reported by Chiodini et al. This report initiated the current interest and controversy about a mycobacterial etiology in Crohn's disease. The hypothesis "Crohn's disease is Johne's disease" did not receive widespread recognition, but has lead to the first multicentered efforts to determine whether or not mycobacteria are associated with Crohn's disease.

The differential diagnosis of inflammatory bowel disease includes intestinal infections and a controversy concentrates on a mycobacterial etiology of Crohn's disease. The hypothesis 'Crohn's disease is Johne's disease' has lead to multicentered efforts to determine whether or not mycobacterial are associated with Crohn's disease. The most active research groups contribute in this book to unravelling this hypothesis and provide the reader with an up-to-date review of the available knowledge.

Chris J.J. Mulder,
Dept. Hepatogastroenterology, Rijnstate Hospital,
PO Box 9555, 6800 TA, Arnhem, The Netherlands

Guido N.J. Tytgat,
Dept. Hepatogastroenterology, Academic Medical Centre,
Meibergdreef 9, 1005 AZ, Amsterdam, The Netherlands

HISTORICAL OVERVIEW AND CURRENT APPROACHES IN DETERMINING A MYCOBACTERIAL ETIOLOGY OF CROHN'S DISEASE

Rodrick J. Chiodini

Mycobacteriology unit, Division of Biological and Medical Sciences, Department of Medicine, Brown University and the Rhode Island Hospital, 593 Eddy Street, Providence, Rhode Island 02903 U.S.A.

Although the earliest descriptions of Crohn's disease are said to date back to the later 1600's to early 1700's (24), they are difficult to sort from other undefined intestinal disorders of that era. Perhaps more realistically, since Crohn's disease and intestinal tuberculosis were confused for years and such confusion continues to this date, the earliest descriptions probably occurred sometime after the discovery of the tubercle bacillus in 1882 (25). Nevertheless, sometime after that period, an intestinal disease was recognized that was similar to intestinal tuberculosis, but acid fast bacilli could not be visualized in tissues or isolated in culture and the characteristic caseous nodules of tuberculosis were absent. By 1913, cases of intestinal tuberculosis which did not fit the classical pattern were well recognized, but nevertheless, were classified among the tuberculous lesions and the disease was known as hyperplastic tuberculosis (44). By the 1920's, these cases of intestinal tuberculosis which did not contain caseous necrosis or acid fast bacilli were reclassified as nonspecific granulomata (30,44) in an attempt to recognize these cases as distinct from the classical or hypertrophic forms of intestinal tuberculosis. Each description, however, discussed the remarkable resemblance of these cases to intestinal tuberculosis - the only difference being the absence of the pathognomonic lesions of tuberculosis, caseous necrosis and acid fast bacilli.

In 1932, the landmark article of Crohn, Ginsberg, and Oppenheimer (14) brought recognition of a disease to be known as regional ileitis as an distinct entity and separated these cases from intestinal tuberculosis. Crohn and his colleagues also recognized the "remarkable resemblance" of their regional ileitis and intestinal tuberculosis. For over 50 years, regional ileitis or Crohn's disease as it is now known, has been regarded as a granulomatous ileocolitis of unknown etiology, distinct from that of intestinal tuberculosis and other mycobacterioses. Unfortunately, identification of the etiology and treatment for patients inflicted with this disorder has progressed little over the last 50 years.

As early as 1826, a chronic enteritis was reported in cattle that could not be associated with any currently known cause of diarrhea (8). The characteristic gross thickening and corrugation of the intestinal mucosa in these animals was recognized, but it was not until 1895 that the etiologic agent was discovered to be an acid fast bacillus (23). At that time, the disease was called pseudotuberculous enteritis, and was thought to be caused by the avian tubercle bacillus (Mycobacterium avium) since the morphologic characters of the organism resembled that species more than Mycobacterium tuberculosis. The name pseudotuberculosis was given to this disease in recognition of its remarkable similarity to intestinal tuberculosis, but without caseous necrosis. However, unlike M. avium or M. tuberculosis, this organism resisted cultivation. It was fifteen years later, in 1910, that Twort (38) succeeded in isolating the causative agent of this disorder. The isolation was largely the result of a laboratory mistake and a perceptive eye for fine detail - Twort noticed small satellite colonies arising around colonies of the common hay bacillus (Mycobacterium phlei) in culture tubes which had inadvertently not been cleaned for several months. It is now known that this organism requires an exogenous growth factor, mycobactin, extracted from other species of the genus and requires at least 3-4 months for laboratory growth (8). The organism was named, at the time, Mycobacterium enteriditis chronicae pseudtuberculosae bovis Johne (39). Between the period of its discovery in 1985 and the isolation of its etiologic agent in 1910, pseudotuberculous enteritis was reported from around the world (8). Over the years, the disease became known as paratuberculosis, commonly as Johne's disease, and in 1932, the organism was officially given the name M. paratuberculosis, although synonyms such as M. johnei were used for years after. Since the discovery of paratuberculosis as a disease, little progress has been made in its diagnosis, control, or treatment. For almost 100 years now, paratuberculosis has been spreading through the world's ruminant domestic livestock and wildlife - it remains difficult to diagnose or control, and no animal has ever been cured (8).

The first suggested connection between Johne's disease and Crohn's disease occurred in 1913 when Dalziel (15) described several cases of enteritis in human which, although resembling intestinal tuberculosis, he believed represented a new disorder. Recognizing the incredible similarity between his cases in humans and those of pseudotuberculosis recently described in cattle, he proposed "that the diseases may be the same". He also recognized a major distinction between these two diseases and expressed a view, still largely held to this date, that "In my cases the absence of acid fast bacilli would suggest a clear distinction...". He felt, however, that the histologic lesions were so similar that it justified his proposition even in the absence of demonstrable acid fast bacilli. Dalziel's views were never given much merit and the classification of these human cases as hyperplastic tuberculosis as proposed by Ingram (44) prevailed. If Dalziel were alive today, ...

Although Crohn and his colleagues (14) ended the dispute of a mycobacterial etiology of the disorder in humans for almost 50 years, a few sporadic individuals failed to accept this general dissassociation and attempted to search for mycobacteria in Crohn's disease. Many, however, did their searching quietly, perhaps in fear of waking an old dead horse. In 1952, van Patter (41), in an effort that remains unpublished except as part of his dissertation, attempted to culture mycobacteria from the intestinal tissues of 43 patients with Crohn's disease. Although reported as a negative study, acid fast organisms which failed to grow on subculture, were isolated from 3 (7%) patients. Further efforts to associate Crohn's disease and mycobacteria took another 25 years to emerge. In 1978, Burnham et al (2) reported the isolation of M. kansasii from the lymph node of a patient with Crohn's disease and pleomorphic variable acid fast organisms from 22 of 27 Crohn's disease patients, 7 of 13 ulcerative colitis patients, and 1 of 11 controls. These investigators proposed that Crohn's disease and ulcerative colitis were caused by cell wall deficient forms of M. kansasii. This hypothesis, however, did not receive widespread recognition and the role of cell wall deficient forms of M. kansasii as etiologic agents in inflammatory bowel disease was short lived. A few of the investigators, although remaining largely in the shadows, continued their efforts and search for a connection between their cell wall deficient organisms and Crohn's disease (37).

In recent years, a variety of different approaches have been used to examine the relationship between mycobacteria and Crohn's disease. These have included cultivation, examination of immune reactivity, animal model studies, anti-mycobacterial treatment, and molecular biology.

CULTURAL STUDIES

In 1984, the isolation of an M. paratuberculosis - like organism from 2 patients with Crohn's disease, but not from 3 patients with ulcerative colitis or 3 with other bowel disorders was reported (9). These isolations were particularly interesting because the organism resembled that which caused a similar and well recognized granulomatous ileocolitis in ruminants known as paratuberculosis (8). It was perhaps this report which initiated the current controversy and which has lead to perhaps the first true concerted effort to determine whether or not mycobacteria are etiologically associated with Crohn's disease. In the last few years, there have been more reports on mycobacteria and Crohn's disease than in the last 100 years or more. This current worldwide effort and excitement (by at least some) over a mycobacterial etiology of Crohn's disease was perhaps generated by 2 unrelated circumstances: 1) the isolation of an organism with a reputation for causing a disease very similar to Crohn's disease in animals; and 2) after 50 years of getting no where, with all theories including autoimmune, dietary, viral, etc., loosing ground, and with medical treatment supportive at best, the time was perhaps right to awaken an old dead horse.

Although the status of investigations of the role of mycobacteria and Crohn's disease has recently been reviewed in detail (4), there have been many achievements in the last few years. These advances have largely been possible by the discovery of IS900, a species specific insertion sequence of M. paratuberculosis (18), and the application of the polymerase chain reaction (PCR) and other molecular approaches. Readers are referred elsewhere for detailed discussions of previous findings (4).

The original studies suggesting an etiologic role of M. paratuberculosis - like organisms in Crohn's disease were expanded, and it was determined that primary isolation of this organism was in the form of a spheroplast or cell wall deficient form (12). These spheroplast-like agents were reported to have been isolated from 16 of 26 patients with Crohn's disease (61%), but not from 13 patients with ulcerative colitis or from 13 patients with other bowel disorders (12). Of these 16 Crohn's disease - associated spheroplasts, 4 had transformed into classical bacillary forms resembling M. paratuberculosis. One of these cultures required 5 years for the emergence of macroscopically visible colonies. By a variety of molecular techniques, including DNA:DNA hybridization (28,45), 5s ribosomal DNA analysis (5,12), and restriction fragment length polymorphism (29), these organisms were definitively identified as M. paratuberculosis. Recently, the remaining 12 unidentified spheroplasts from the Crohn's disease patients and several from controls were examined by PCR for the presence of IS900. An additional 6 cultures from Crohn's disease patients were identified as containing M. paratuberculosis, bringing the total number of isolates from these investigators to 10 out of 26 or 38% of all Crohn's disease cultures (42). IS900 was not detected in any culture from non - Crohn's disease sources.

In addition to these initial investigators, others have participated in searching for mycobacteria in Crohn's disease patients. In Australia, Dr. P. Coloe of the Royal Melbourne Institute of Technology isolated M. paratuberculosis from a patient with Crohn's disease, representing the first group to reproduce earlier findings. Other isolations soon came from France, California, Houston, and The Netherlands (4). Dr. G. Gitnick at the University of California in Los Angeles, isolated a strain of M. paratuberculosis from 1 of 27 patients with Crohn's disease, but not from 29 patients with ulcerative colitis or 26 with other bowel disorders (17); although other Mycobacterium spp. were isolated from ulcerative colitis, control, and Crohn's disease cultures. Other investigators have also attempted cultivation, but their efforts are less defined and the reader is referred elsewhere for these discussions (4).

At present, the 3 most active groups attempting to culture mycobacteria from Crohn's disease patients are Chiodini, who's efforts have largely already been described above, D. H. Graham from the Baylor College of Medicine, and J. Haagsma of the Veterinary Research Institute in The Netherlands.

Graham and coworkers (26) initially reported a vast number of mycobacterial isolates from Crohn's disease patients (5 of 59 or 15%), ulcerative colitis patients (9 of 19 or 47%), and non-IBD controls (18 of 27 or 67%). Most of these isolated were environmental Mycobacterium spp., primarily Mycobacterium avium and Mycobacterium fortuitum. In addition to these bacillary forms, these investigators also isolated spheroplast or assumably cell wall deficient variable acid fast organisms, primarily from Crohn's disease tissues. Examination of these unidentified spheroplast forms revealed the presence of IS900 (M. paratuberculosis) in 6 of 18 (33%) Crohn's disease cultures examined, in none of 6 ulcerative colitis cultures, and in only 1 of 5 non-IBD controls (31).

Haagsma et al (19) cultured tissues from 100 patients with Crohn's disease and 50 from patients with ulcerative colitis or other intestinal disorders. Of the 100 Crohn's disease cultures, approximately 50 have been lost to contamination by other microbes and were considered unsuitable for evaluation. Of the remaining 50 Crohn's disease cultures, they have been successful in isolating M. paratuberculosis from 10 of them, but not from any of their ulcerative colitis or other control tissues (32). In addition, this group has been successful in identifying acid-fast bacilli from an additional 10-15 patients, but these have not been identified as yet.

In summary, of the 3 major groups involved in cultivation of mycobacteria from Crohn's disease, M. paratuberculosis has been isolated or otherwise detected in culture from 38%, 33%, and 20% out of a total of approximately 135 patients, but from only 1 of over 121 non-Crohn's disease controls. This sort of distribution suggests more than a casual role for this organism in the etiology of Crohn's disease.

One of the major complications to our understanding of the role of these organisms in Crohn's disease is the widespread distribution of mycobacteria in the environment which complicate not only the isolation of particular species, but also our interpretation of their isolation. As we learn more about this particular organism and that of closely-related environmental species, we may begin to understand the role of mycobacteria in Crohn's disease.

GENETIC STUDIES

As discussed earlier, the application of molecular biology to the study of mycobacteria in Crohn's disease and the discovery of IS900 in M. paratuberculosis, has resulted in major advances in our understanding of the distribution of M. paratuberculosis and its possible association with Crohn's disease (20).

Initially, these methods were used to determine the identification of these M. paratuberculosis - like agents from Crohn's disease tissues, and by a variety of methods including DNA:DNA hybridization, analysis of 5s ribosomal DNA genes, and restriction fragment length polymorphisms, these organisms were definitively identified as M. paratuberculosis (5,28,29). Recently, by examination of RFLP of IS900, it was further determined that the human isolates resemble those of cattle strains more than those obtained from ovine or caprine species (13,43). These findings suggest that the source or reservoir of these organisms in humans may be the domestic cattle population.

The two major advances accomplished by molecular biology has been the use of PCR in combination with IS900 to examine unidentified cultured organisms and the direct examination of tissues for the presence of this sequence.

Many investigators referred to above and many addressed previously (4), had been successful in isolating unidentified organisms from tissues of both Crohn's disease patients and controls, but the slow growth of these organisms precluded their identification by conventional methods. It has not in the past been possible to intelligently speak of these isolates because their identity was unknown, and even if mycobacterial in origin, the widespread distribution of mycobacteria in the environment preclude any suggestions related to etiologic or pathogenic potentials. The discovery of IS900 (18) as a species-specific marker of M. paratuberculosis allowed for the first time the ability to specifically identify this species. Combined with the amplification of PCR, a powerful tool emerged. Examination of unidentified cultures from Crohn's disease and controls revealed IS900 in 38% (10 of 26) of Crohn's disease cultures in one study (42) and in 33% (5 of 15) in another (31), thereby suggesting that about 1/3 of cultures from Crohn's disease patients have detectable levels of M. paratuberculosis. Based on the hybridization signals, it has been estimated that these cultures contained between 3 and 30 individual mycobacterial cells (genomes) per culture pellet. Such results suggest that these strains either fail to grow in vitro or grow at an extremely slow rate. Using a more ubiquitous probe against the 65 Kd heat shock protein, mycobacterial sequences of unknown species were detected in Crohn's disease as well as control cultures (42), again illustrating the ubiquitous nature of mycobacteria in general and the need to define your objectives and organisms at the species level.

Another application of molecular biology has been the direct detection of mycobacterial DNA in tissue specimens. Earlier studies using DNA:DNA hybridization techniques to search for mycobacteria in Crohn's disease patients were complicated by the large number of hybridizations suggesting the presence of mycobacterial DNA in 53% (10 of 19) of Crohn's disease biopsies, 33% (2 of 6) of ulcerative colitis patients, and

17% (1 of 6) of normal controls (45). These results were comparable to studies on the environmental distribution of mycobacteria and suggested increased colonization of mycobacteria in Crohn's disease. Without the ability to differentiate species, these findings had little etiologic meaning.

With IS900, the ability to specifically search for this species was possible and PCR provided the sensitivity needed to detect an organism that was below the detection level of acid-fast light microscopy or immunohistochemistry. Application of PCR and IS900 to biopsy specimens revealed the presence of M. paratuberculosis in 65% (26 of 40) of Crohn's disease patients, 4.3% (1 of 23) of ulcerative colitis patients, and 12.5% (5 of 40) of non-IBD controls (35). These findings have several important implications. The finding of IS900 in controls indicates a previously unrecognized environmental distribution of this organism, suggesting that environmental contact with M. paratuberculosis may be common. The low presence of M. paratuberculosis in ulcerative colitis patients suggest that colonization of the disrupted or abnormal intestinal mucosa by M. paratuberculosis does not occur. Therefore, the high prevalence in Crohn's disease patients would suggest some etiologic role. A casual relationship between IS900 and Crohn's disease is not supported by these studies as a similar distribution should have been observed in ulcerative colitis.

IMMUNOLOGY

Immunologic studies on the reactivity of Crohn's disease patients to mycobacterial antigens have been sparse and inconclusive, and the reader is referred elsewhere for a review of previous efforts (4). In general, patients with Crohn's disease fail to elicit any consistent humoral or cell mediated response to mycobacterial antigens. Although we and others have observed some responsiveness, the results are generally not reproducible (4). While superficially these findings would suggest an etiologic dissassociation between Crohn's disease and mycobacteria, the nature of the studies performed do not provide a solid framework on which to reach that conclusion.

The pathologic lesion of Crohn's disease, in general, can be considered a delayed type hypersensitivity type reaction resembling a tuberculoid lesion. By definition, such a lesion is mediated by cellular elements of immunity which may not be accompanied by a humoral response. Therefore, the absence of any demonstrable humoral response to mycobacterial antigens in Crohn's disease would not be unexpected. On the other hand, one would expect a cellular response to mycobacterial antigens in Crohn's disease if these agents were etiologically related. No such response, however, has been consistently demonstrated. There may be several reasons for such, few of which have been adequately examined.

Crohn's disease is a mucosal disease and the sequestered nature of the lesions suggest that effector cells may be compartmentalized within the intestine. Therefore, examination of peripheral reactivity may not be appropriate. There are multiple examples in chronic infectious diseases, including mycobacterial, in which vigorous responses can be demonstrated in infected tissues in the absence of peripheral activity (33,36). Cases with extraintestinal lesions may be the only cases in which humoral reactivity might be expected.

Additionally, and perhaps more importantly, the widespread reactivity of the general population to environmental antigens (1,16) may preclude detection of a specific response. In our studies of peripheral reactivity to mycobacterial antigens in Crohn's disease by a lymphocyte blastogenesis assay (unpublished observation), most Crohn's disease patients responded well to M. paratuberculosis antigens. However, despite a strong response by the Crohn's disease patient group, it was not significantly different from the control population. The response of the control group was so high that a specific response in Crohn's disease would not have been demonstrated even if such existed. It is not a case that Crohn's disease patients do not respond, but rather that their response cannot be differentiated from normal responses.

Current evidence suggests that if mycobacteria are causative agents in Crohn's disease that they exist in an altered form, probably as a spheroplast or other pleomorphic form without a full cell wall. Under such conditions, the antigens present and expressed may be quite different from those found in the bacillary form since most of the immunogenic antigens are cell wall associated. Therefore, to find a specific response in Crohn's disease patients, it may be necessary to look at reactivity of specific antigens in order to separate specific responses from those obscured by general environmental reactivity. In tuberculoid leprosy, for example, humoral reactivity to M. leprae is generally not demonstrable unless specific antigens, such as PGL-1, are used and only then can specific antibody responses be detected (34). Unfortunately, few specific antigens currently exist for M. paratuberculosis.

In consideration of immunologic reactivity, one must also consider statistical data which in itself may preclude the detection of immune reactivity. There is considerable debate on whether or not Crohn's disease is a single disease entity. Regardless of the position one wishes to hold, most will agree that the characteristics of Crohn's disease are ambiguous enough that it could comprise several etiologies. If we assume cultural and molecular biology data to represent the possible infection rate with M. paratuberculosis, i.e., 65% or less; recognize the inconsistency in detection of immune reactivity in most chronic infections, e.g., compartmentalization, anergy, etc.; the effects of contact with the agent by nonsusceptible hosts; and then add a 20% diagnosis error as suggested by epidemiologic studies (3); a consistent immunologic response in Crohn's disease to its etiologic agent, what ever it might be, would be difficult to detect. This is not to imply that investigations are not warranted or unlikely to show cellular reactivity to mycobacteria, but rather to bring to light that such studies may begin with many lines drawn against success.

ANIMAL MODEL STUDIES

There have been several attempts by various investigators to develop mycobacterial models of Crohn's disease, but in this authors opinion, none have been particularly successful. Our initial studies in goats (40) do not provide an appropriate model in many respects because, although a natural host of M. paratuberculosis, the disease is of the lepromatous form rather than a tuberculoid disease as seen in humans. Even in the disease observed in primates (27), the lesions and corresponding immune reactivity is lepromatous. Since Crohn's disease, regardless of its etiology, clearly has a major immunologic component, comparison between tuberculoid and lepromatous disease is not entirely appropriate since different immunologic mechanisms exist. To compare tuberculoid to lepromatous leprosy is like comparing apples and oranges.

This putative agent, M. paratuberculosis, does not readily infect species other than ruminants (8). To accomplish such generally requires modulation of the immune response which may destroy the animal as an appropriate model. Can a disease which contains a major immunologic component as the disease causing factor itself be successfully studied in an immunodeficient or immunocompromised host? While meaningful data can be derived from such studies, they do not represent realistic models in which to study pathogenesis.

For years investigators have sought animal models of paratuberculosis but none has been found to be appropriate (8). The same seems likely with Crohn's disease. It may be necessary to explore other animals but their cost may not offer the advantage generally dictating animal models. For instance, the disease observed in subhuman primates (stumptail macaques) was of the lepromatous form, but we were unsuccessful in infecting other subhuman primates (rhesus). Other primates, however, may be susceptible and provide a tuberculoid-type disease, but their cost and per diem charges would likely preclude their use over human clinical studies.

If mycobacteria are ultimately found to be involved in the pathogenesis (or perhaps more appropriately immunopathogenesis) of Crohn's disease, animal models are likely to play a major role in determining certain aspects of the disease process.

TREATMENT

There have been numerous studies on the efficacy of treatment of Crohn's disease with various antimicrobial (anti-mycobacterial) agents, but few have been scientifically valid enough to draw any conclusive conclusions (see 4 for review). There are a large number of case reports suggesting efficacy of anti-mycobacterial chemotherapy in Crohn's disease, but to date, no controlled study has shown any conclusive (objective) benefit of such treatment. The reasons for such failures may be based on the manner in which these studies were conducted, and unfortunately, continue to be conducted. No animal with M. paratuberculosis infection has ever been cured.

We have learned over the years that one cannot extrapolate data from the treatment of tuberculosis to leprosy, or visa versa, or to other mycobacterial infections. Even within the Enterobacteriacae, it is known that effective therapy with one species does not necessarily provide efficacy with infection by another. Therefore, the choice of treatment regimes based on tuberculosis may be inappropriate. In recent years we have gained a great deal of knowledge in the treatment of M. avium infections, in both compromised and non-compromised patients, and such data would perhaps be more appropriate to base treatment regimes. Alternately, or concurrently, susceptibility patterns for M. paratuberculosis strains isolated from Crohn's disease patients have been determined for single drugs and multiple combinations (6,7,11) and should be considered. It must, however, be appreciated that in vitro effects and therapeutic efficacy may not always agree, particularly with regard to intracellular organisms.

Current advances in the treatment of M. avium pulmonary infections in non-immunocompromised patients suggests that at least 3 or more drugs need to be used simultaneously and continued for 3.6 +/-0.5 years in order to achieve clinical improvement (21). In light of these findings, the use of single or double anti-mycobacterial drugs in the treatment of Crohn's disease for a 6-month period would seem rather inadequate. It must be appreciated that all antimicrobial agents work only during the replicative phase of bacterial growth - these agents have no effect during stationary or other nonproliferative state. According to all data accumulated to date, if mycobacteria, particularly M. paratuberculosis, are involved in the pathogenesis of Crohn's disease, they exist within the intestine in very small numbers and in a form which rarely replicates. Under such a situation, the 3.6 years required for M. avium infections may not be long enough to eliminate M. paratuberculosis and its antigens should they exist in Crohn's disease.

Furthermore, there exists the possibility that a 6-month limited drug trial could make the patient transiently worse rather than better. As an immunologically based disease (like most mycobacterial infections) the killing of organisms with their subsequent release of antigens could conceivably cause a worsening of symptoms, perhaps similar to the reversal reaction in leprosy (22). It must also be appreciated that intestinal tuberculosis cannot be cured by chemotherapy alone but require surgical intervention.

In summary, to conclusively evaluate the efficacy of anti-mycobacterial chemotherapy in Crohn's disease, the use of multiple drug combinations for extended periods need to be evaluated. The statistical matters discussed under immunology will also need to be considered in patient selection and analysis of data.

CONCLUSIONS

Progress over the last few years regarding the role of mycobacteria in Crohn's disease have not progressed as fast as many may have anticipated or wished. There are various reasons for the slow progress. If Crohn's disease is caused by M. paratuberculosis or another Mycobacterium spp., it is not the classical picture of tuberculosis or leprosy, but some unique unusual manifestation which is not fully understood. The classical mycobacterioses have puzzled scientist for well over 100 years and something outside this picture is going to be even more difficult to understand. Pathogenic mycobacteria elicit one of the most complex, and in many respects most poorly understood, immunological events known. After all, disease by these organisms is caused by the host's response to them rather than any effect they cause on the host. Understanding the classical diseases are difficult enough; novel approaches will be required to understand a non-classical disease.

There are also a limited number of investigators actively studying this particular subject and funding is in general sparse. As a result, progress has been, and will likely continue to be, slow. Increased efforts are likely to be limited until the controversy surrounding this issue subsides and mycobacteria become convincingly established as etiologic agents in at least some cases of Crohn's disease.

Although there are various aspects of Crohn's disease as related to mycobacteria that are perhaps needed to be understood, the primary objective must be in establishing a definitive role for these agents in Crohn's disease. Aspects unrelated to this primary objective will have little meaning unless an etiologic role is firmly established. Unfortunately, differing views exist, largely because there are no clear cut answers and a variety of approaches will be required to collectively provide a determination. At present, the greatest hope lies in molecular biology and the demonstration of etiologic agents directly in tissues. These techniques are most likely to provide the strongest evidence of an association and these studies are currently in progress. The other major area, since Crohn's disease contains a major immunologic component, is identification of the antigenic determinant(s) and immunologic responses that are giving rise to the chronic inflammation. These may be unique antigens or antigens cross-reactive with mucosal tissue. Reactivity may also be associated only within the intestinal lymphoid cells. There is general agreement that if mycobacteria are etiologically related to Crohn's disease, a cellular response must be present and that response will need to be demonstrated in addition to the demonstration of mycobacteria in tissues.

In summary, there has been a great deal of effort since 1984 investigating the role of mycobacteria, specifically M. paratuberculosis, as etiologic agents in Crohn's disease. The data suggesting a role is largely based on cultural isolation or other methods of detection of a well known animal pathogen from the tissues of Crohn's disease patients, but interpretation of the data has been complicated by the isolation of closely related environmental mycobacteria from both Crohn's disease patients and controls. Nevertheless, it is now conclusively and irrefutably shown that M. paratuberculosis can be found within the tissues of a major proportion of Crohn's disease patients. With current studies and efforts continuing, this association is likely to become more and more established and the etiologic role of M. paratuberculosis in Crohn's disease will likely gain momentum.

As methods are improved and an understanding of the environmental distribution of mycobacteria is achieved, the significance of these pathogenic strains will become more evident. Although it has been a slow path down the road, recent advances suggest an answer to this intriguing and controversial subject may be approaching in the near future.

The old horse isn't dead yet and current evidence may even suggest that it is not only being revived, but may be nursed into good health.

REFERENCES

1 Bermudez LEM, Wu M, Enkel H, et al. Naturally occurring antibodies against Mycobacterium avium complex. Ann Clin Lab Sci 1989;19:435-443.

2 Burnham WR, Lennard-Jones JE. 1978. Mycobacteria as a possible cause of inflammatory bowel disease. Lancet 2693-696.

3 Calkins BM, Mendeloff AI. 1986. Epidemiology of inflammatory bowel disease. Epidemiol. Rev. 8:60-91.

4 Chiodini RJ. 1989. Crohn's disease and the Mycobacterioses: a review and comparison of two disease entities. Clin. Microbiol. Rev. 2:90-117.

5 Chiodini RJ. 1990. Characterization of Mycobacterium paratuberculosis and organisms of the Mycobacterium avium complex by restriction polymorphism of the rRNA gene region. J. Clin. Microbiol. 28:489-494.

6 Chiodini R J. 1990. Bacteriocidal activity of various antimicrobial agents on human and animal isolates of Mycobacterium paratuberculosis. Antimicrob. Agents Chemother. 34:366-367.

7 Chiodini RJ. 1991. Antimicrobial synergism of rifabutin in combination with other antimicrobial agents against strains of Mycobacterium paratuberculosis. J. Antimicrob. Chemother. 27:171-176.

8 Chiodini RJ, Van Kruiningen HJ, Merkal RS. 1984. Ruminant paratuberculosis (Johne's disease): The current status and future prospects. Cornell Vet. 74:218-262.

9 Chiodini R J, Van Kruiningen HJ, Merkal RS, Thayer WR, Coutu JA. 1984. Characteristics of an unclassified Mycobacterium species isolated from patients with Crohn's disease. J. Clin. Microbiol. 20:966-971.

10 Chiodini RJ, Van Kruiningen HJ, Thayer WR, Merkal RS, Coutu JA. 1984. The possible role of mycobacteria in inflammatory bowel disease. I. An unclassified Mycobacterium species isolated from patients with Crohn's disease. Dig. Dis. Sci. 29:1073-1079.

11 Chiodini RJ, Van Kruiningen HJ, Thayer WR, Coutu JA, Merkal RS. 1984. In vitro antimicrobial susceptibility of a Mycobacterium species isolated from patients with Crohn's disease. Antimicrob. Agents Chemother. 26:930-932.

12 Chiodini RJ, Van Kruiningen HJ, Thayer WR, Coutu JA. 1986. The spheroplastic phase of mycobacteria isolated from patients with Crohn's disease. J. Clin. Microbiol. 24:357-363.

13 Collins DM, Gabric DM, de Lisle GW. 1990. Identification of two groups of Mycobacterium paratuberculosis strains by restriction endonuclease analysis and DNA hybridization. J. Clin. Microbiol. 28:1591-1596.

14 Crohn B, Ginzburg L, Oppenheimer G. 1932. Regional ileitis, a pathological and clinical entity. JAMA 99:1323-1329.

15 Dalziel TK. 1913. Chronic interstitial enteritis. Br. Med. J. 2:1068-1070.

16 Edwards LB, Acquaviva FA, Livesay VT et al. An atlas of sensitivity to tuberculin, PPD-B, and histoplasmin in the United States. 1969; 99(Suppl):1-132.

17 Gitnick G, Collins J, Beaman B, Brooks D, Arthur M, Imaeda T. 1988. Prospective evaluation of mycobacterial infection in Crohn's disease: isolation and transmission studies. In: Inflammatory Bowel Disease. Current status and future approach. (R. P. MacDermott, Ed.) Excerpta Medica,Elsevier Science Publ. Co., Amsterdam. pp. 527-534.

18 Green EP, Tizard MLV, Moss MT, Thompson J, Winterbourne DJ, McFadden JJ, Hermon-Taylor J. 1989. Sequence and characteristics of IS900, an insertion element identified in a human Crohn's disease isolate of Mycobacterium paratuberculosis. Nuc. Acid Res. 17:9063-9073.

19 Haagsma J, Mulder CJJ, Eger E, Bruins J, Ketel RJ, Tytgat GNJ. 1988. Mycobacterium species isolated from patients with Crohn's disease. In: Inflammatory Bowel Disease. Current status and future approach. (R. P. MacDermott, Ed.) Excerpta Medica, Elsevier Science Publ. Co., Amsterdam. pp. 535-538.

20 Hermon-Taylor J, Moss M, Tizard M, Malik Z, Sanderson J. 1990. Molecular biology of Crohn's disease mycobacteria. Ball. Clin. Gastroenterol. 4:23-42.

21 Hornick DB, Dayton CS, Bedell GN, Fick RB. 1988. Nontuberculous mycobacterial lung disease. Substantiation of a less aggressive approach. Chest 93:550-555.

22 Imkamp FM. 1985. Standardized schemes for steroid treatment in ENL and reversal reactions. Int. J. Lepr. Other Mycobact. Dis. 53:313-317.

23 Johne HA, Frothingham L. 1895. Ein eigenthuemlicher Fall von tuberkulose beim Rind. Dtsch. Ztschr. Tiermed. Path. 21:438-454.

24 Kirsner JB. 1982. The "idiopathic" inflammatory bowel diseases. Their cause and pathogenesis. Arch. Dermatol. 118:280-282.

25 Koch R. 1882. Die aetiologie der tuberculose. Berlinger Klinische Wochenschrift 19:221-230.

26 Markesich DC, Graham DY, Yoshimura HH. 1988. Progress in culture and subculture of spheroplasts and fastidious acid-fast bacilli isolated from intestinal tissues. J. Clin. Microbiol. 26:1600-1603.

27 McClure HM, Chiodini RJ, Anderson DC, Swenson RB, Thayer WR, Coutu JA. 1987. Mycobacterium paratuberculosis (Johne's disease) in a colony of stumptail macaques Macaca arctoides). J. Inf. Dis. 155:1011-1019.

28 McFadden JJ, Butcher PD, Chiodini RJ, Herman-Taylor J. 1986. Determination of genome size and DNA homology between an unclassified Mycobacterium species isolated from patients with Crohn's disease and other mycobacteria. J. Gen. Microbiol. 133:211-214.

29 McFadden JJ, Butcher PD, Chiodini RJ, Hermon-Taylor J. 1987. Crohn's disease-isolated mycobacteria are identical to Mycobacterium paratuberculosis, as determined by DNA probes that distinguish between mycobacterial species. J. Clin. Microbiol. 25:796-801.

30 Moschcowitz E, Wilensky A. 1923. Nonspecific granulomata of the intestine. Am. J. Med. Sci. 166:48-66.

31 Moss MT, Sanderson JD, Tizard MLV, Hermon-Taylor J, El-Zaatari F, Markesich D, Graham DY. Identification of M. paratuberculosis by PCR in long term cultures of Crohn's disease tissue. Proc. 3rd Intl. Colloq. Paratb., Orlando, Florida; Sept 28-Oct 2, 1991. In press.

32 Mulder CCJ. 1991. personal communication.

33 Rook GAW, Carswell JW, Stanford JL. 1976. Preliminary evidence for the trapping of antigen-specific lymphocytes in the lymphoid tissue of 'anergic' tuberculosis patients. Clin. Exp. Immunol. 26:129-132.

34 Saad MH, Medeiros MA, Gallo ME, Gontijo PP, Fonseca LS. 1990. IgM immunoglobulins reacting with the phenolic glycolipid-1 antigen from Mycobacterium leprae in sera of leprosy patients and their contacts. Mem. Inst. Oswaldo. Cruz 85:191-194.

35 Sanderson JD, Moss MT, Tizard MLV, Hermon-Taylor J. 1992. PCR detection of Mycobacterium paratuberculosis in Crohn's disease tissue DNA extracts. Proc. 3rd Intl. Colloq. Paratb., Orlando, Florida; Sept 28-Oct 2, 1991. In press.

36 Schlossman SF, Levin HA, Rocklin RE, David JR. 1971. The compartmentalization of antigen-reactive lymphocytes of desensitized guinea pigs. J. Exp. Med. 134:741-750.

37 Stanford JL, Dourmashkin R, McIntyre G, Visuvanathan S. 1988. Do mycobacteria exist in alternative physical forms and what part may they play in the aetiology of inflammatory bowel disease. In: Inflammatory Bowel Disease. Current status and future approach. (R. P. MacDermott, Ed.) Excerpta Medica, Elsevier Science Publ. Co., Amsterdam. pp. 503-508.

38 Twort FW. 1911. A method for isolating and growing the lepra bacillus of man and the bacillus of Johne's disease in cattle (preliminary note). Vet. J. 67:118-120.

39 Twort FW, Ingram GLY. 1912. A method for isolating and cultivating the Mycobacterium enteritidis chronicae pseudotuberculosae bovis, Johne and some experiments on the preparation of a diagnostic vaccine for

pseudotuberculous enteritis of bovines. Proc. Roy. Soc. Ser. B84:517-542 [also in Vet. J. 68:353-365].
40 Van Kruiningen HJ, Chiodini RJ, Thayer WR, Coutu JA, Merkal RS, Runnels PL. 1986. Experimental disease in infant goats induced by a Mycobacterium from a patient with Crohn's disease. Dig. Dis. Sci. 31:1351-1360.
41 Van Patter WN. 1952. Pathology and Pathogenesis of regional enteritis. Ph.D. dissertation, University of Minnesota.
42 Wall S, Soufleri I, Seechurn P, Saboor S, Chiodini R, McFadden JJ. 1992. Identification of spheroplast-like agents isolated from Crohn's disease and control tissues using the polymerase chain reaction. J. Clin. Microbiol. Submitted.
43 Whipple D, Kapke P, Vary C. 1990. Identification of restriction fragment length polymorphisms in DNA from Mycobacterium paratuberculosis. J. Clin. Microbiol. 28:2561-2564.
44 Wilensky A, Moschcowitz E. 1927. Nonspecific granulomata of the small intestine. Am. J. Med. Sci. 173:374-380.
45 Yoshimura HH, Graham DY, Estes MK, Merkal RS. 1987. Investigation of association of mycobacteria with inflammatory bowel disease by nucleic acid hybridization. J. Clin. Microbiol. 25:45-51

MYCOBACTERIAL ISOLATES FROM CROHN'S DISEASE IN THE NETHERLANDS.

Jan Haagsma[1], Chris J.J. Mulder[2] and Anthony Eger[1], Guido N.J. Tytgat[3]

1 Central Veterinary Institute, Dept. of Bacteriology, Lelystad, The Netherlands.
2 Rijnstate Hospital, gastroenterologist, Arnhem, The Netherlands.
3 Academic Medical Centre, Amsterdam, The Netherlands.

INTRODUCTION

After the first publication of Chiodini et al (1984) a joint study was started in order to investigate the role of mycobacteria, in particular of M. paratuberculosis, in the etiology of Crohn's Disease. In the Central Veterinary Institute research on paratuberculosis is going on for more than 30 years and bacteriology has always been an important item.
Thousands of specimen have been examined for the presence of M.paratuberculosis and the standard isolation procedure is as follows:
After grinding, in particular faeces and intestinal tissue need a decontamination treatment in order to prevent the contamination of the media with other bacteria and fungi.
We are using a combination of 4% sodium hydroxide followed by 5% oxalic acid (Beenwerth, 1967), each 15 minutes. Three different media (Loewenstein modified, Stonebrink and Ogawa) are used and per specimen always 6 slants are inoculated.
M.paratuberculosis needs a special growth factor, the so-called mycobactin, which regulates the transport of iron through the cell-wall. This mycobactin is produced by other mycobacteria and we incorperate the widely used product from M.phlei. Recently, some researchers have suggested that mycobactin J from M.paratuberculosis might give slightly better results. In our hands the difference is doubtful and therefore we still use phlei-mycobactin. Moreover, we know since some years that strain M18 which is used for the production of mycobactin J is not M.paratuberculosis but a M.avium strain. The sensitivity of our isolation procedure is very good, up to 10 bacteria per gram faeces or tissue can be detected. The joint study has been focused on the isolation of M.paratuberculosis from CD patients, not on other mycobacterial species.

MATERIALS AND METHODS

Several modifications were introduced in order to be as sure as possible that technical failures in the isolation procedure could not be responsible for negative results. These modifications resulted in a very comprehensive isolation procedure.

- **Grinding**

The first modification concerns the grinding of the specimen: Besides the high speed rotation of the omnimixer, a more gentle grinding was carried out in 60% of the samples in a mortar with sand and pestle, in order to avoid mechanical damage of more sensitive bacterial forms.

- **Decontamination**

The decontamination was also modified. From 1984-1986 the same procedure as for cattle was used, namely 15 min. 4% NaOH followed by 5% oxalic acid.
Since 1986 only oxalic acid was used and the time was shortened to 5 min., because in contrast to cattle samples, the number of contaminated slants from human samples was very low and again we wanted to be sure that this procedure should not harm less vital bacteria.
Besides oxalic acid, also HPC (hexadecylpyridium chloride) was used, although in our cattle samples 0,75% HPC gave disappointing results.

- **Mycobactin**

Another modification concerns the mycobactin. Besides the mycobactin P used in our standard procedure for cattle, mycobactin P as whole phlei-bacteria and mycobactin J were also used. Negative controls were always included.

- **Media**

Table 1 shows the various media and the number of slants which has been used. Own experience and from colleagues abroad has shown that various M.paratuberculosis strains may have different nutrient requirements.

F.i. isolates from sheep and goat in Spain (Juste, 1991) grow significantly better on media without pyruvate in contrast with normal cattle strains.
So we tried to cover the different requirements in order to be as sure as possible that the composition of the media could not be responsible for negative results.
Moreover, inoculating so many slants (32, but Coletsos was omitted since 1988) means that more tissue material is used for examination, resulting in a higher isolation chance.

TABLE 1 **Isolation media for CD-patients**

Medium	Number of media
L/J	5
Ogawa	5
Stonebrink	7
Herolds Egg Yolk	6
Smith/Dubos	5
Middlebrook 7H10	2
Coletsos (1984-1988)	2
	—
Total	32

Modifications:	+ and - mycobactin	(resp. 24 and 8 slants)
	+ and - pyruvate	(resp. 12 and 20 slants)
	+ and - antibiotics	(resp. 14 and 18 slants)

- **Origin of the specimen**

Specimen from 112 patients have been examined, 97 from CD, 5 from Colitis Ulcerosa and 10 controls with other diseases from the intestinal tract (Table 2).

TABLE 2 **Patient specimen (N=112)**

	Intestinal Surgery*	tissue Biopsy	Intestine + Lymphnode	Lymphnode	Total
Crohns's Disease	54	11	31	1	97
C.U.	3	1	1		5
Controles	10				10
	—	—	—	—	—
	67	12	32	1	112

* full-thickness intestine, resection specimen.

From 65 CD patients only intestinal tissue was available, 54 times resection specimen with full-thickness intestine and 11 times biopsy tissue. From 31 CD patients, both intestine + regional lymph node were received and from 1 patient only the lymph node.
From Colitis Ulcerosa cases the same tissues were examined but from controls only intestinal tissue.

RESULTS

The study started in September 1984 with 2 small biopsy samples obtained via the University of Leiden, and from 1 sample M. paratuberculosis was isolated.

Stimulated by this success we have examined since December 1985 95 CD specimen and in 2 other patients M. paratuberculosis was demonstrated.
The 5 Colitis Ulcerosa cases and 10 controls are negative so far.

Table 3 shows that the incubation period of the cultures varies between less than 6 months and more than 2 years. Most samples have passed 2 years incubation.

In the three positive cases growth of M. paratuberculosis was observed within 1 year.

If no growth of colonies is observed after 2 years, all slants, even if no suspicious spots are seen, are harvested with a minimum of saline. From the turbid suspension a Ziehl-Neelsen stain is performed and the rest is transferred to 7 fresh media (2 LJ, 2St, 2 Ogawa and 1 Middlebrook 7H10). The Ziehl-Neelsen stain showed weak acid fast rods in 3 cases, and pleomorphic forms which were partly weak acid fast, in 20 cases (Table 3). Colonies indicating bacterial growth have not been observed on the fresh media, of the second passage except in 1 interesting case. This case concerned pleomorphic forms collected from slants from patient H. from with M. paratuberculosis was already isolated after 3 months.
From the pleomorphic forms a subculture with M. paratuberculosis colonies was obtained after 8 months. These observations demonstrate that these pleomorphic forms and rods might be important, but that other technics are necessary for identification, f.i. DNA probes and the use of a specific PCR.

In Table 4 more detailed information concerning our 3 M. paratuberculosis isolates is presented.

In our first case (patient V) from intestinal biopsy tissue, growth of colonies was observed after a long incubation period of 11 months on Herrolds egg yolk, and after 13 months on the Ogawa egg based medium. The decontamination procedure was different; in one isolate the standard procedure for cattle samples was used (NaOH and oxalic acid) and in the other isolate 0,75% HPC. In our second case (patient H) from colon tissue growth of colonies was obtained after the relative short incubation period

of 3 months on Middlebrook 7H10 and only after 17 months on LJ. These isolates were obtained both after grinding in an omnimixer and in a mortar which is more suitable for small specimen (f.i. biopsies).
And in all positive media mycobactin from M. phlei was included, so no positive results with mycobactin J were obtained.

TABLE 3 Results of bacteriological examination

	Incubation in months 0 - 6	6 - 12	12 - 18	18 - 24	>24
M. paratuberculosis	1	2	0	0	0
Acid fast rods	-	-	-	-	3
Acid fast pleomorphs	-	-	-	-	20*
Negative	5	10	4	3	64

* Including isolate H., subculture pos. after 8 months.

TABLE 4 M. paratuberculosis isolates

Patient	Year	Incubation	Medium	Decontam.	Grinding	Myc.
V.	1984	a 11	Herrold	NaOH+Ox	mortar	phlei
		b 13	Ogawa	HPC	mortar	phlei
H.	1988	a 3	7H10	Ox	omnimixer	phlei
		b 17	L/J	Ox	omnimixer	phlei
M.	1989	a 6*	L/J	Ox	omnimixer	phlei

* Contaminated culture (with M. fortuitum)
Identification by DNA-hybridization (H. Taylor)

The isolates were identified as M. paratuberculosis by the cultural and biochemical properties and this identification was confirmed by DNA-DNA hybridization.

The third isolate (patient M.) is a more complicated story because a mixed growth occurred of a rapid grower and a slow grower resembling M. paratuberculosis.

The rapid grower could be obtained in pure culture and identified as M. fortuitum.
However, due to overgrowth, it was impossible to get a pure culture from

the slow grower.

The mixed culture has been send in 1989 to Dr. Herman Taylor in London and he was able to identify the slow grower as M. paratuberculosis by the PCR with M. paratuberculosis specific IS 900 primers.

CONCLUSIONS

1 Despite comprehensive isolation procedures M. paratuberculosis was isolated only in 3 out of 97 CD cases.
2 There was not a distinct preference for one of the various modifications of our isolation procedure.
3 Weak acid fast rods and pleomorphic forms have been found in 23 cases but it was impossible to transfer this material to growth of colonies.
4 Further identification of these forms might help to elucidate the role of M. paratuberculosis in the etiology of C.D.
Addendum: Very recently 5 samples with pleomorphic forms were examined in cooperation with Herman Taylor and Moss (St. Georges Hospital, London) by the PCR with M.para- tuberculosis specific IS900 primers and in 3 samples the presence of M. paratuberculosis DNA could be demonstrated. Further research with more samples is going on.
5 The 15 non CD control samples are negative so far.
6 Final remark: There is smoke but we can not yet identify the fire.

REFERENCES

- Beerwerth, W. 1967. Die Züchtung von Mykobakterien aus dem Kot der Haustiere und ihre Bedeutung für die Epidemiologie der Tuberkulose. Prax Pneumol 21;189-202.

- Chiodini RJ, van Kruiningen HJ, Merkal RS, Thayer WR and Contu JA. 1984. Characteristics of an unclassified Mycobacterium species isolated from patients with Crohn's disease. J Clin Microbiol 20;966-971.

- Juste RA, Marco JC, de Ocariz CS and Aduriz JJ. 1991. Comparison of different media for the isolation of small ruminant strains of Mycobacterium paratuberculosis. Vet Microbiology 28;385-390.

ATTEMPTS AT CULTURING MYCOBACTERIA FROM TISSUES OF PATIENTS WITH CROHN'S DISEASE

Georg Kreuzpaintner*, Richard Kölble*, Axel Wallner*, Rudolf Hesterberg+, Marie Francoise Thorel°, Lutz Thomas#, Georg Strohmeyer*

* Departments of Gastroenterology, + Surgery and # Medical Microbiology and Virology, Heinrich-Heine-University Düsseldorf, Düsseldorf, Germany

° Laboratoire Central de Recherches Vétérinaires, Maisons-Alfort Cedex, France

ARGUMENTS FOR A MYCOBACTERIAL ETIOLOGY IN CROHN'S DISEASE

Since the description of regional enteritis by Crohn, Ginzburg and Oppenheimer (1) in 1932 only the report of Burnham et al. (2) drew attention to a mycobacterial etiology in Crohn's disease. In 1978 he isolated Mycobacterium kansasii from one mesenteric lymph node and cell-wall-deficient organisms from 81 % of mesenteric lymph nodes obtained from patients with Crohn's disease. A mycobacterial etiology in Crohn's disease was revived by the detection of Mycobacterium paratuberculosis in Crohn's disease in 1984 (3). Chiodini found Mycobacterium paratuberculosis in the mucosa of patients with Crohn's disease in 15.4 % and in addition cell-wall-deficient organisms in 46.2 % (4) whereas all controls remained negative. These data are the basis for the connection of Crohn's disease with Johne's disease (5) in veterinary medicine. Johne's disease is a chronic granulomatous and wasting disease of ruminants caused by Mycobacterium paratuberculosis. Both Crohn's disease and Johne's disease show remarkable similarities which make them indistinguishable in clinic, epidemiology and pathology (6).

At present a mycobacterial etiology in Crohn's disease is supported by:

1. The international isolation of Mycobacterium paratuberculosis in 10 patients with Crohn's disease.
2. A successful therapy with tuberculostatics in Crohn's disease in most trials and case reports.
3. The detection of specific IgG directed to the common 45/48 kilodalton doublet antigen of Mycobacterium tuberculosis, Mycobacterium avium and Mycobacterium paratuberculosis in 65 % of patients with Crohn's disease.
4. The more frequent detection of genomes specific for Mycobacterium paratuberculosis in tissues and long term cultures of patients with Crohn's disease compared to controls.

In the meantime Mycobacterium paratuberculosis has been isolated from six additional patients with Crohn's disease round the world (7-9), but not in controls (Table I).

TABEL 1 Isolates of Mycobacterium paratuberculosis from patients with Crohn's disease

Investigator	Country	Number of isolates/ number of patients	Isolates	Year
Chiodini	USA	4/26	15.4 %	1984-86
Haagsma	The Netherlands	3/97	3.1 %	1985-89
Coloe	Australia	1/30	3.3 %	1986
Gitnick	USA	1/27	3.7 %	1989
Thorel	France	1/nk*		1989

* nk: not known

Antituberculous therapy was effective in 53.9 % of 76 Crohn's disease patients refering to all case reports and trials (n = 11) reported (10-20) (Table II). Because antimycobacterial drugs have been selected randomly for these trials the drug regimens varied from a monotherapy with rifampicin or dapsone to a quadruple drug therapy with pyrazinamide, rifampicin, isoniazid and ethambutol, and were performed 2 - 24 months.

TABEL II Antimycobacterial chemotherapy in Crohn's disease

Investigator	Year	Patients n	Number of tuberculostatics applied n	Duration (months) n	Therapeutic effect %
Ward	1975	6	1	> 3	67
Schaffer	1984	14	2	24	0
Warren	1986	1	4 (2)	2 (7)	100
Wirostko	1987	4	1	11-18	100
Schultz	1987	1	4 (3)	2 (2)	100
Hampson	1988	17 (5)	4 (5)	6	71
Rutgeerts	1988	10	2	6	0°
Thayer	1988	12	2 (1)	2-4 (>2-4)	100
Picciotto	1988	1	3	9	100⁺
Järnerot	1989	5	4	8-13	80#
Prantera	1989	5	1	2-12	40

* Two yaer randomised double blind, crossover, placebo controlled trial.
° No improvement of the lesions in the neoterminal ileum at endoscopy.
⁺ Relapse after 9 months under antimycobacterial chemotherapy.
Relapse of 2 patients (40 %) after 12 and 13 months under antimycobacterial chemotherapy.

The only randomised, double blind, crossover, placebo controlled trial used rifampicin and ethambutol for a period of two years. Only 14 Crohn's disease patients completed the trial which revealed no significant effect of the antimycobacterial drugs on the course of the underlying disease (11). The second negative trial used exclusively endoscopic criteria for the estimation of therapeutic effectiveness (17). Only studies which used rifabutin in combination with an aminoglycoside or quadruple therapy showed improvement in patients with Crohn's disease following antimycobacterial chemotherapy (16, 18, 19).

General guidelines for the treatment of pulmonary mycobacterioses include at least quadruple drug therapy and treatment durations of two to three years. Until now no study fulfils these requirements. Therefore, data on the efficacy of antimycobacterial chemotherapy in Crohn's disease are needed on the basis of its effectiveness in atypical mycobacteria, multiple drug regimens, long term administration and sufficient patient numbers.

A mycobacterial etiology in Crohn's disease is further supported by the detection of specific IgG directed to the common 45/48 kilodalton doublet antigen of Mycobacterium tuberculosis, Mycobacterium avium and Mycobacterium paratuberculosis in 65 % of sera obtained from patients with Crohn's disease compared to 0 - 10 % in controls. This immunoblot assay developed by Pranab K. Das (21) possess a specificity of about 80 - 90 % and a sensitivity of 65 % for patients with Crohn's disease.

Molecular biology provides strong evidence for the increased presence of genomes specific for Mycobacterium paratuberculosis in tissues of patients with Crohn's disease compared to controls. After enzymatic extraction from full thickness samples of surgically resected intestine polymerase chain reaction for Mycobacterium paratuberculosis was performed using oligonucleotide primers amplifying a 400 base pair portion of the 5' -region of IS900, a multicopy genomic DNA insertional element highly specific for this organism. One Mycobacterium paratuberculosis genome could be detected in the reaction. Mycobacterium paratuberculosis was detected in 26 of 40 Crohn's disease patients (65 %), but only in 4 of 27 controls (14.8 %) (22). Surprisingly these data are quite similar as compared to the results of the immunoblot assay detecting specific IgG directed to a common mycobacterial doublet antigen (see above). The same investigators examined also long term cultures of resected intestinal tissue as well as of endoscopic mucosal biopsy with the same polymerase chain reaction assay. Mycobacterium paratuberculosis was present in 6 of 18 patients with Crohn's disease (33.3 %), but only in 1 of 11 controls (9.1 %) (23) (see also Professor J. Hermon-Taylor, this symposiumbook).

The isolation of Mycobacterium paratuberculosis only from patients with Crohn's disease by Chiodini (3, 4) stimulated us to reproduce these results in a non veterinary laboratory. Compared to the methods applied by Chiodini the specimens were processed immediately and the decontamination period of mucosa was reduced from 18 till 24 hours to 50 minutes. In addition two mesenteric lymph nodes and one serosa slice removed during surgery were investigated.

MATERIALS AND METHODS

- **Patients**

Tissues of 22 patients who underwent intestinal resection for Crohn's disease (11 male, 11 female; mean age + SD, 30.5 + 10.9 years (yr); range, 13-62 yr) were investigated for fastidious, mycobactin-dependent mycobacteria. The diagnosis of Crohn's disease had been established by clinical criteria as well as X-ray, endoscopy, and histology. In 2 patients only colon, in 6 patients only small intestine, and in 14 patients the large and small bowel were involved. The average duration of disease was 8.5 + 5.8 yr (range, 1.5-26.4 yr).

Up to several weeks prior to and at the time of surgery 10 patients received systemic corticosteroids, 6 fluocortolone (range, 10-50 mg/day), 2 methylprednisolone (12-16 mg/day), 1 prednisone (20 mg/day), 1 hydrocortisone (5-25 mg/day), and 1 additional betamethasone enema (2.5 mg/day). Eight patients received salazosulfapyridine (2-3 g/day), 5 patients 5-aminosalicylic acid (1.5 g/day) (1 additionally 750 mg/day as suppository), 5 antibiotics, 4 cefotaxime (6 g/day), 3 metronidazole (1.25-1.5 g/day), and 1 trimethoprim-sulfamethoxazole (0.32 g/1.6 g/day); six patients were on parenteral nutrition. Ileum was resected in 3 patients, small and large bowel in 19 patients. Fistulae (range, 1-6) were removed in 13 patients, abscesses (range, 1-3) in 5 patients. The disease activity was assessed by Crohn's disease activity index (CDAI) (24) which averaged 321 + 165 (x + SD; range, 86-679). In 4 patients (18.2 %) the CDAI was < 150.

- **Controls**

Tissues of 22 patients with other diseases of the colon (15 adenocarcinomas, 2 ulcerative colitis, 3 diverticulosis, 1 diverticulitis, 1 tubular adenoma; 8 male, 14 female; mean age + SD, 62.1 + 16.1 yr; range, 25-79 yr) served as controls. The diagnoses were made by established clinical, radiologic, endoscopic and histopathologic criteria. In 2 patients with ulcerative colitis the disease had been present for 3 months and 6 years and 7 months, respectively. Before surgery both received fluocortolone 40 and 60 mg/day, one additionally salazosulfapyridine (3 g/day), parenteral prednisolone (75 mg/day) and parenteral nutrition, the other metronidazole (1.2 g/day). The disease activity was determined using the score of Rachmilewitz (25) which amounted to 13 and 4 in the patients with ulcerative colitis, representing severe and moderately severe illness according to Truelove and Witts (26). Colon was resected in all 22 patients, the terminal ileum in 9. In both patients with ulcerative colitis 1 or 2 fistulae were removed.

- **Collection and processing of specimens**

During surgery 2 mesenteric lymph nodes and 1 serosa slice were removed from the resected intestine. In 1 patient with Crohn's disease and 2 controls no lymph nodes were harvested and in 1 patient with Crohn's disease no serosa was obtained. About one third of the lymph nodes was used for histological examination. A small metastasis was detected in 1 lymph node from a patient with adenocarcinoma. All patients except one control with diverticulosis and allergy to antibiotics received antibiotics immediately before or during surgery in addition to the medication mentioned above. In Crohn's disease the patients received 2 g moxalactam alone (20x), or combined with 0.5 g metronidazole (3x), the controls 2 g moxalactam (19x), 2 g cefotaxime and 0.5 g metronidazole (1x), or 1.2 g amoxicillin (1x). However, 13 patients with Crohn's disease and 17 controls had not received any antibiotic before the removal of the 2 lymph nodes and the serosa slice. The surgeon left the surgical specimen in a sterile plastic bag for transport to the Pathology Department, where it was cleaned with sterile 0.9 % (wt/vol) NaCl and sections were removed for histologic examination under aseptic conditions using sterile gloves, instruments and operative towels as well as a surgical mask.

Remaining tissues were rewrapped in a new sterile plastic bag and immediately transported to the Institute for Medical Microbiology and Virology for immediate processing under sterile conditions using a Gelaire BSB 4 (Flow Laboratories Ltd., Meckenheim), sterile gloves, instruments, glass-ware and material. The lymph nodes were trimmed of fat and minced as well as the serosa slice. Further trituration was achieved by grinding with a glass homogenizer (model Eppendorf, Braun, Melsungen). After digestion with 10 ml sterile 2.5 % (wt/vol) trypsin (1:250, Difco Laboratories, Detroit, MI) in phosphate buffer (66.7 mmol/l, pH 7.5) (Merck, Darmstadt) for 30 min with continuous stirring at room temperature, the lymph nodes and the serosa slice were centrifuged at 4419 g for 30 min in sterile polypropylene tubes (Becton Dickinson, Lincoln Park, NJ). Thereafter 1 lymph node of each patient was decontaminated with 10 ml 0.1 % (wt/vol) benzalkonium chloride (Merck) for 10 min and centrifuged at 4419 g for 5 min. If visible contamination had occured during surgery both lymph nodes and the serosa slice were decontaminated for 10-30 min.

In each patient 10 g mucosa were prepared and triturated. In addition mucosa was harvested from another part of the intestine if available, e.g. from both small and large bowel or jejunum and ileum. The weight of the additional mucosa preparation ranged between 1.39 and 10 g in Crohn's disease, and between 0.7 and 10 g in the controls. In Crohn's disease mucosa of jejunum (n = 2), ileum (n = 20) and colon (n = 16) was investigated, in the controls from ileum (n = 6) and colon (n = 22). 10 g prepared mucosa were placed into 10 ml of the trypsin solution, dispersed with 20 000 rpm for 30 s using a dispersive apparatus (Ultra-Turrax T25, S25N-18G, particle size 10-50 μm, Janke & Kunkel, Staufen), and digested with 40 ml trypsin with continuous stirring for 30 min. During digestion the pH was corrected with sterile 1 N NaOH (Merck). Lesser amounts of mucosa were digested with 10 or 20 ml trypsin. After digestion larger particles of tissue were removed by filtration through a sterile metal tea-strainer with a mesh size of 0.5 mm followed by centrifugation at 4419 g for 30 min in polypropylene tubes. The resulting sediment of mucosa was suspended in 40 ml sterile 0.1 % benzalkonium chloride. After trituration with forceps, scissors, scalpel and a glass homogenizer 0.25 g mucosa as well as about 10 % of each lymph node and serosa were suspended in hypertonic Middlebrook 7H9 medium (Difco) without trypsin digestion.

- **Media and incubation**

Middlebrook 7H9 medium was prepared as described (27) containing 2 mg/l mycobactin J (Allied Laboratories Inc., Glenwood Springs, CO). Hyperosmolarity was achieved with 20 % (wt/vol) filtered (pore size 220 nm) (Millipore, Eschborn) glucose (Difco) in final concentration. The homogenate was passed through a filter with a pore size of 220 nm into Falcon tissue culture flasks (Becton Dickinson). 50 ml (25 cm2) tissue culture flasks contained 7.5 ml homogenate from each lymph node or serosa, each of two 250 ml (75 cm2) tissue culture flasks contained 22.5 ml from one mucosa. The tissue culture flasks were incubated at 37°C in a horizontal position in accordance with a medium depth of about 3 mm without agitation. Filtered hypertonic Middlebrook 7H9 medium alone served as negative control.

Herrold egg yolk medium was prepared fresh every 5 weeks using hen eggs free of antibiotics. 1020,2 ml Herrold egg yolk medium contained 9.0 g peptone, 15.3 g Noble agar, 2.7 g beef extract, 2.25 g asparagine, 27.0 ml glycerol, 5.1 ml 2 % (wt/vol) malachite green (Difco), 2 mg mycobactin J (4.0 ml), 4.5 g NaCl (Merck), 874.1 ml sterile and double distilled water minus x ml 1 N NaOH, and 110.0 ml egg yolk harvested under aseptic conditions. Half of the media were improved with 4.1 g sodium pyruvate (Boehringer, Mann-heim). After stirring, pH 7.2 was adjusted with sterile 1 N NaOH followed by the addition of mycobactin J and sterilisation for 25 min at 121°C and 1 bar. Sterile malachite green was added followed by homogenised egg yolk, stirring, and distribution of the medium into slanted test tubes.

To prevent contamination in long term cultures we avoided to work with Mycobacterium paratuberculosis in our institution. Therefore from each preparation four slants of Herrold egg yolk medium two containing pyruvate were sent to Dr. M. F. Thorel, Laboratoire Central de Recherches Veterinaires, Paris, and served as positive controls. There the

slants were inoculated with the subculture of Mycobacterium paratuberculosis 7912, a strain isolated from a bull (n = 36), or a wild strain of Mycobacterium paratuberculosis (n = 32). A concentration of bacilli of 1 mg/ml was used.
After allowing the suspended mucosa to stand in benzalkonium chloride for 50 min at room temperature, each of 8 slants of Herrold egg yolk medium (half containing pyruvate) were inoculated with 100 μl of the resulting sediment. After centrifugation the sediment of lymph nodes and serosa was suspended in 1.3 ml of nutrient broth (Difco), pH 7.2, which was prepared as described (27) and contained additionally 4.588 g NaCl, 0.68 g Na_2HPO_4 (Merck), 2.25 g asparagine, 2 ml glycerol and 2 mg mycobactin J per liter. Eight slants of Herrold egg yolk medium (half containing pyruvate) were inoculated with each tissue (100 μl). The tubes were locked with Barthmann plugs and incubated at 37°C. Four slants of Herrold egg yolk medium, two containing pyruvate, served as negative controls by inoculation with 100 μl each of 0.9 % NaCl, nutrient broth, trypsin or benzalkonium chloride.
Cultures were examined weekly for the first month, thereafter monthly. Aerobic contaminants were detected by subculture on blood-agar plates. No attempt was made to detect anaerobes.
Subcultures were performed on Herrold egg yolk medium containing pyruvate and in Middlebrook 7H9 medium supplemented with 10 % (vol/vol) oleic-albumin-glucose-catalase (Becton Dickinson), 0.05 % (vol/vol) Tween 80 (Difco), and 2 mg/l mycobactin J, or 10 % (vol/vol) Dubos oleic albumin complex (Becton Dickinson), 0.05 % (vol/vol) Tween 80, and 2 mg/l mycobactin J.

RESULTS

In order to prevent damage to mycobacteria by the decontamination with benzalkonium chloride, the decontamination period of the mucosa was reduced from 18 - 24 hours as reported by Chiodini to 50 minutes. Lymph nodes and serosa were decontaminated only for 10 minutes, if at all. 60 % of lymph nodes and serosa were not decontaminated. In addition, lymph nodes and serosa had been removed before the application of antibiotics in 62 % of patients with Crohn's disease and 77 % of controls.
Control media with or without pyruvate enabled very good or good growth, respectively, of Mycobacterium paratuberculosis strain 7912 or a wild strain after 4 - 6 weeks of incubation. Only one Herrold egg yolk medium (1.5 %) inoculated with strain 7912 showed no growth. All negative controls remained without growth.

The mean incubation period of the cultures was 841 + 130 days (x + SD), range 382 - 1055 days, in Crohn's disease and 648 + 194 days (x + SD), range 372 - 1046 days, in controls. No growth was found in hypertonic Middlebrook 7H9 medium. Gram stain and Ziehl-Neelsen stain of this broth revealed no bacteria or bacterial material.

However, after an average incubation period of 11.9 months small translucent colonies with a diameter of approximately 0.5 mm were detected on Herrold egg yolk media of 9 patients with Crohn's disease. In addition whitish colonies were found in the cultures of two patients with Crohn's disease. Allover growth was obtained from 10 patients with Crohn's disease (45.5 %) of 15 different tissues (Table III). No growth was observed in controls.

Ziehl-Neelsen stain of primary colonies yielded different results (Table III): Acid-fast masses were found in a colony isolated from the mesenteric lymph node of one patient with Crohn's disease. In two patients Ziehl-Neelsen stain revealed acid-fast bodies among amorphous material. Acid-fast and non-acid-fast coccoid bodies among amorphous material were found in 10 different tissues of 7 Crohn's disease patients. Ziehl-Neelsen stain of whitish colonies revealed acid-fast and non-acid-fast coccoid bodies in one case and non-acid-fast coccobacilli in the other. Ziehl-Neelsen stain of culture material from controls was negative. Gram stain, so far performed, was negative in Crohn's disease patients and controls.

DISCUSSION

Contamination with mycobacteria was excluded with greatest possible security as these investigations were performed in a virologic laboratory of the Institute for Medical Microbiology where never had been worked with Mycobacterium paratuberculosis or other mycobacteria until now. Therefore a contamination of our cultures with mycobacteria is impossible. In addition, our Herrold egg yolk media were examined in the Laboratoire Central de Recherches Veterinaires in Paris and yielded good to very good growth of Mycobacterium paratuberculosis.

After an average incubation period of 11.9 months a very scarce growth of small, mostly translucent colonies was detected on Herrold egg yolk medium only in patients with Crohn's disease. In spite of subcultivation on Herrold egg yolk medium and in supplemented Middlebrook 7H9 medium we did not succeed in the transformation from spheroplast to bacillary state till now. Ziehl-Neelsen stain revealed a pleomorphic picture which reached from acid-fast masses to non-acid-fast coccobacilli (Table III). All Gram stains were negative. Allover we found growth in 45.5 % of patients with Crohn's disease, however in no control. The extremely slow growth only on this special culture medium for Mycobacterium paratuberculosis and the staining behaviour suggest cell-wall-deficient forms, most likely of a mycobacterium of Runyon group III to which also belongs Mycobacterium paratuberculo-

TABEL III Cultural and microscopic data of Herrold egg yolk medium in Crohn's disease and controls

		Growth after months		in Patients		from Tissues	Lymph node	Serosa	Colonic mucosa	Ileal mucosa	Controls
	x ± SD	Minimum	Maximum	n	%	n	n	n	n	n	n
Primary culture	11.9±6.8	4.6	21.4	10	45.5	15	6	4	2	3	0
Translucent colonies	11.1±6.9	4.6	21.4	9	40.9	13	6	3	2	2	0
Whitisch colonies	16.9±1.6	15.8	18.0	2	9.1	2		1		1	0
Ziehl-Neelsen stain											
Acid-fast mass	5.5			1	4.5	1	1				0
Acid-fast coccoid bodies among amorphous material	6.5±2.1	5.0	8.0	2	9.1	2	1			1	0
Acid-fast and non-acid-fast coccoid bodies among amorphous material	12.6±7.3	4.6	21.4	7	31.8	10	4	3	2	1	0
Acid-fast and non-acid-fast coccoid bodies	15.8			1	4.5	1				1	0
Non-acid-fast coccobacilli	18			1	4.5	1		1			0

sis. Further investigations for detection of L-forms as well as the identification of the organism by transformation and/or polymerase chain reaction are required and are already at work to some extent.

Burnham had isolated cell-wall-deficient organisms in 81 % from mesenteric lymph nodes of Crohn's disease patients, in 54 % of patients with ulcerative colitis, and 9 % of patients without inflammatory bowel disease (2). Only in one mesenteric lymph node (4 %) of Crohn's disease patients he found Mycobacterium kansasii. Stanford isolated pleomorphic variable acid-fast organisms from mesenteric lymph nodes of 42 of 76 Crohn's disease patients (55 %), 14 of 27 ulcerative colitis patients (52 %), and 3 of 41 controls (7 %) (28). Exclusively in patients with Crohn's disease Chiodini found in 61.6 % cell-wall-deficient bacilli, from which he could transform 15.4 % into Mycobacterium paratuberculosis (3, 4). Smears from biopsy specimens revealed acidfast bacilli in 11 of 32 patients with active Crohn's disease (34 %), but not in controls (29). Mycobacterium chelonei was isolated from two patients with active Crohn's disease. Visuvanathan (M.D. thesis) isolated extremely slow growing pleomorphic acid-fast organisms from mesenteric lymph nodes of 17 of 25 patients with Crohn's disease (68 %), 11 of 15 ulcerative colitis patients (73 %), and 3 of 17 controls (18 %) (30). Cell-wall-deficient forms were less frequently isolated by Haagsma from 6 of 97 patients with Crohn's disease only (6.2 %) (7), by Gitnick from 2 of 27 patients with Crohn's disease (7.4 %) which were transformed and identified as Mycobacterium chelonei subspecies abscessus and Mycobacterium paratuberculosis (8), and by Graham from 12 of 59 Crohn's disease patients (20.3 %), 3 of 19 patients with ulcerative colitis (15.8 %), but not from controls (31). Our data with the exclusive detection of pleomorphic, variable acid-fast organisms in 45.5 % of Crohn's disease patients are in line with most of these data reported and support a possible etiologic role of mycobacteria or their cell-wall-deficient forms in Crohn's disease.

REFERENCES

1 Crohn BB, Ginzburg L, Oppenheimer GD. Regional ileitis. A pathologic and clinical entity. JAMA 1932;99:1323-1329.

2 Burnham WR, Lennard-Jones JE, Stanford JL, Bird RG. Mycobacteria as a possible cause of inflammatory bowel disease. Lancet 1978;2:693--696.

3 Chiodini RJ, Van Kruiningen HJ, Thayer WR, Merkal RS, Coutu JA. Possible role of mycobacteria in inflammatory bowel disease. I. An unclassified Mycobacterium species isolated from patients with Crohn's disease. Dig Dis Sci 1984;29:1073-1079.

4 Chiodini RJ, Van Kruiningen HJ, Thayer WR, Coutu JA. Spheroplastic phase of mycobacteria isolated from patients with Crohn's disease. J Clin Microbiol 1986;24:357-363.

5 Morgan KL. Johne's and Crohn's. Chronic inflammatory bowel diseases of infectious aetiology? Lancet 1987;1:1017-1019.
6 Chiodini RJ. Crohn's disease and the mycobacterioses: a review and comparison of two disease entities. Clin Microbiol Rev 1989;2:90-117.
7 Haagsma J, Mulder CJJ, Eger A, Tytgat GNJ. Mycobacterium paratuberculosis isolated from patients with Crohn's disease. Preliminary Dutch results. Acta endoscopica 1991;21:2:255-260.
8 Gitnick G, Collins J, Beaman B, Brooks D, Arthur M, Imaeda T, Palieschesky M. Preliminary report on isolation of mycobacteria from patients with Crohn's disease. Dig Dis Sci 1989;34:925-932.
9 Coloe PJ, Wilks CR, Lightfoot D, Tosolini FA. Isolation of a Mycobacterium species resembling M. paratuberculosis from the bowel tissue of a patient with Crohn's disease (abstract). Aust Microbiol 1986;7:188.
10 Ward M, McManus JPA. Dapsone in Crohn's disease (letter). Lancet 1975;1:1236-1237.
11 Shaffer JL, Hughes S, Linaker BD, Baker RD, Turnberg LA. Controlled trial of rifampicin and ethambutol in Crohn's disease. Gut 1984;25 :203-205.
12 Warren JB, Rees HC, Cox TM. Remission of Crohn's disease with tuberculosis chemotherapy (letter). N Engl J Med 1986;314:182.
13 Wirostko E, Johnson L, Wirostko B. Crohn's disease. Rifampin treatment of the ocular and gut disease. Hepato-gastroenterol 1987; 34: -90-93.
14 Schultz MG, Rieder HL, Hersh T, Riepe S. Remission of Crohn's disease with antimycobacterial chemotherapy (letter). Lancet 1987;2: 1-391-1392.
15 Prantera C, Argentieri R, Mangiarotti R, Levenstein S. Dapsone and remission in Crohn's disease (letter). Lancet 1988;1:536.
16 Hampson SJ, Parker MC, Saverymuttu SH, McFadden JJ, Hermon-Taylor J. Results of quadruple antimycobacterial chemotherapy in 17 Crohn's disease patients completing six months treatment (abstract). Gastroenterology 1988;94:A170.
17 Rutgeerts P, Vantrappen G, Van Isveldt J, Geboes K. Rifabutin therapy in patients with recurrent Crohn's disease after ileocolonic resection (abstract). Gastroenterology 1988;94:A391.
18 Thayer WR, Coutu JA, Chiodini RJ, Van Kruiningen HJ. Use of rifabutin and streptomycin in the therapy of Crohn's disease (abstract). Gastroenterology 1988;94:A458.
19 Järnerot G, Rolny P, Wickbom G, Alemayehu G. Antimycobacterial therapy ineffective in Crohn's disease after a year (letter). Lancet 1989;1:164-165.
20 Prantera C, Bothamley G, Levenstein S, Mangiarotti R, Argentieri R. Crohn's disease and mycobacteria: two cases of Crohn's disease with high anti-mycobacterial antibody levels cured by dapsone therapy. Biomed Pharmacother 1989;43:295-299.
21 Das PK, Blaauwgeers JLG, Slob AW, Yong SL, Rumbukkanna A. Mycobacterial antibody (Myc-Ab) response in relation to Crohn's disease (CD) (abstract). Gastroenterology 1989;96:A111.

22 Sanderson JD, Malik Z, Moss MT, Tizard MV, Green EP, Hermon-Taylor J. Polymerase chain reaction (PCR) directly reports Mycobacterium paratuberculosis (M.para) genomes in Crohn's disease tissue DNA extracts (abstract). Gastroenterology 1991;100:A247.

23 Moss MT, Sanderson JD, Tizard MV, Hermon-Taylor J, El-Zaatari F, Markesich DC, Graham DY. Mycobacterium paratuberculosis (M. para) in long term cultures of Crohn's disease tissue revealed by PCR amplification of IS900 (abstract). Gastroenterology 1991;100:A232.

24 Best WR, Becktel JM, Singleton JW, Kern F Jr. Development of a Crohn's disease activity index. Gastroenterology 1976;70:439-444.

25 Rachmilewitz D. Coated mesalazine (5-aminosalicylic acid) versus sulphasalazine in the treatment of active ulcerative colitis: a randomised trial. Br Med J 1989;298:82-86.

26 Truelove SC, Witts LJ. Cortisone in ulcerative colitis: final report on a therapeutic trial. Br Med J 1955;2:1041-1048.

27 Difco Manual. Dehydrated culture media and reagents for microbiology. 10th ed. Detroit: Difco Laboratories, 1984.

28 Stanford JL. Acid fast organisms in Crohn's disease and ulcerative colitis. In: Pena AS, Weterman IT, Booth CC, Strober W, editors. Recent advances in Crohn's disease. The Hague: Martinus Nijhoff, 1981:274-278.

29 Colemont LJ, Pattyn SR, Michielsen PP, Pen JH, Pelckmans PA, Van Maercke YM, Portaels F. Acid-fast bacilli in Crohn's disease (letter). Lancet 1988;1:294-295.

30 Visuvanathan S. The characterisation of pleomorphic acid fast organisms isolated from patients with inflammatory bowel disease (dissertation). London: University of London, 1991.

IMMUNOHISTOLOGICAL EVIDENCE FOR MYCOBACTERIA IN CROHN'S DISEASE

Pranab K. Das[1,2], Ada W. Slob[2], Arnold Stronkhorst[3], Sander J.H. van Deventer[3] and Guido N.J. Tytgat[3].

Departments of Dermatology(1), Pathology(2) and Gastroenterology(3)
Academisch Medisch Centrum, University of Amsterdam.
The Netherlands.

INTRODUCTION

Despite an enormous amount of investigations the etiology of Crohns disease (CD) remains unknown. Exogenous factors, both of non infectious (e.g. food) and infectious (bacteria and virus) agents have been often postulated as the causatives (1-3).

Nevertheless, results of controversial studies kept on appearing in literature which often suggested that the granulomatous disease may sometime be induced in animals by inoculating tissue filtrates of the diseased gut from CD patients (4-9).

However, inspite of the lack of convincing evidence for the infectious agents as the causatives, investigators continued to relate the disease with some sort of latent infections. In this latter category it was interesting to note that
Dalziel(10) drew attention to the similarity between pseudotuberculosis in cattle (infection by <u>M. paratuberculosis</u>, now known as Johne's disease) and chronic tuberculosis - like enteritis in humans but as a new disease entity. By contrast, Ignard (11) classified this disease as hyperplastic tuberculosis. In later years, due to lack of evidence for the presence of acid-fast bacilli or caseous necrosis, the land mark article of Crohn et al (12) established regional ileitis as a separate non-tuberculosis disease entity.

It is now known that both hypertrophic intestinal tuberculosis and tuberculosis with either caseation or demonstrable acid fast bacilli do exist. Consequently "a mycobacterial etiology" for Crohn's disease attrackted a renewed attention (13-15) and isolated mycobacterial (Myc) species from CD-guts have been mentioned regularly as likely candidates for the causative agent for the disease. However, the culture data on

Myc-species remained controversial (16-19), at least their significance as primary pathogens (20).

PRESENT IMMUNOHISTOLOGICAL STUDY

A General Background

The controversy about the mycobacterial etiology for Crohn's disease (CD) reflects the difficulties either in demonstrating significant presence of mycobacterial organisms or mycobacterial degradation products, in lesional guts and the failure to demonstrate significant host immune response to any dominant mycobacterial antigens (21-26). Further, the increasing molecular evidence for the importance of microbial mimicry antigens (antigens shared between hosts and microorganisms) in autoimmune diseases adds to confusions (27).

Recently, Rook and Stanford contended that several diseases that are thought to be "autoimmune" or "idiopathic" including Crohn's disease are caused by inflection with related mycobacteria (28).

Since mycobacteria are common environmental agents, it is not surprising either to encounter some sequistered mycobacterial residues in the gut or to observe host immunity to certain mycobacterial immunocross reactive antigenic component (Im CRAC). In order to appreciate the significance of these responses a brief understanding of some aspects of mycobacterial ImCRAC induced immunity in mycobacterioses is needed.

B Mycobacterioses and immunopathology

The immunopathology of granuloma's induced by opportunistic mycobacteria has been extensively studied in Leprosy as the model disease (29). From such studies it is evident that sensitisation with mycobacteria can cause different host immune response. Depending on the types of immune responses, the clinical spectra in mycobacterioses can vary from (a) no symptoms/or transient symptoms; (b) diffuse inflammatory mycobacterioses with bacillary load such as lepromatous leprosy (L-lep); self healing mycobacterioses with no demonstrable bacilli(paucibacillary) such as tuberculoid leprosy (T-lep); and intermediate type often with the presence of acid-fast bacilli as an unstable group such as borderline leprosy (B-lep).

This latter group can progress either towards the Polar type I (L-lep) or to Polar type II (T-lep) during the evolution or progress of the disease. The spectral pathology in mycobacterioses is regarded to involve (i) differing immune responses to different groups of mycobacterial Im-CRAC and (ii) differing immunoregulation by both different exogenous inflammatory cytokines e.g. tumour necrosis factors (Tnf-α), interferon (Inf-) and interleukins (Il)(30-31). It is now well recognised that degraded inert components of mycobacteria e.g. peptidoglycolipid, phenolic glycolipid are both potent inflammatory and immunomodulating agents, whereas mycobacterial protein antigens are widely cross reactive, species non restricted and strong immunogens, which can evoke both cell mediated (CMI) as well as humoural (antibody:Ab) responses in a host. Since mycobacteria are environmental agents, it is not surprising that the population at large possess both Ab and CMI to different mycobacterial antigens with or without strain restrictions.

If mycobacteria play a role in the pathogenesis of CD, one would expect that both intact mycobacteria and their degraded products are likely to be detected within inflammatory tissues, such as in inflammatory gut, at certain stages of the diseases. Detection of either mycobacterial degradation products in the diseased bowel or demonstation of an abnormal mycobacterial specific immune response in CD patients would, therefore, be a significant step forward in the reach for "mycobacterial actiology" in CD.

C Aim of the Present Study

The present study was undertaken to provide evidence by immunohistological and other relevant immunological methods for (a) relationships between gut associated mycobacterial antigen(s) and inflammation in CD pathology; and (b) association between immune responses of patients with CD to certain group of mycobacterial Im-CRAC in CD pathology as disease markers.

D Experimentals

1 Test specimens

The following patients' materials were used for immunohistological investigations: (a) surgical resection specimens of terminal ileum and colon from 15 CD, 15 patients with ulcerative colitis (UC), 15 patients with colon cancer (CC), 15 patients with diverticulitis (DC) and relevant control tissues; (b) serum samples from above mentioned specimens as well as patients with tuberculosis and leprosy and from normal healthy controls;

2 Immunohistological methods

Panels of mouse monoclonal antibodies (mAbs) and rabbit polyclonal antibodies (pAbs) with differing specificities to various mycobacterial species Mycobacterium avium (m.av.),
M.bovis BCG, M.tuberculosis and M.leprae and other non-mycobacterial strains were used either by three or two step immuno-peroxidase single staining method on cryostat sections of gut tissues which were pre-fixed by methanol-aceton and air dried.

In addition, double staining methods were also applied using a panel of mAbs to B-cells, T-cells, macrophages, cell activation markers (MHC-class II antigens) and pAbs to immunoglobulin isotypes in combination with the positively reacting mycobacterial antibodies. The immunohistological staining procedures are the same as those described in various publications from our laboratories (32-33). When positive reaction with any of the Abs to bacterial stain were observed, the specific reactivity was strictly controled by both antigen excess inhibition and appropriate elution methods.

3 Relevant Immunological Methods

(Serology: Immunoblotting and ELISA)

Immunoblotting and ELISA of serum antibodies using either subcellular fractions of M.tuberculosis, M.avium, M.bovis BCG and M.paratuberculosis or the specific antigenic components isolated by a preparatory sodium dodecylsulfate polyacrylamide gel electrophoresis (SDS-PAGE) were carried out by the method described by us previously (34,35).

RESULTS AND DISCUSSION:

- Immunohistological Data

After examining a panel of both mAbs and pAbs to mycobacteria and other bacteria, we observed that only two mAb F85-2/F85-10 to specific peptidoglycolipid (pgl) of M.avium (m.av) with common serotype (36), stained a number of cells in gut tissue. By applying an antigen excess inhibition we could establish that the immunostaining was mAb pgl specific. In CD patients, the mean number of these positively stained cells (containing pgl-antigen) were $54\pm$sd25 in comparison to $25\pm$sd9 in UC and $12\pm$sd3 in others and the positively stained were distributed in lamina propria. However, positive reactions were also found on histologically normal gut specimens. Only in CD patients a considerable number of mAbs-pgl stained cells were also found in submucosa and subserosa. Using double staining methods, it was found that the localisation of such m.a.v. - pgl-antigen appeared to be on a particular subset of CD19+, IgA+ or IgG+ or IgM+ B-cells.

Although these anti-mycobacterial antibody reactive subsets were also present in non CD tissues, they were present in lesser numbers and in a different distribution pattern

(37,38). The immunodoublestaining showed that m.a.v. pgl-antigen predominantly localised on IgA+ B-cells and to a lesser extent on either IgG+ or IgM+ B-cells. Further, immunodoublestaining showed that these m.a.v. pgl-bound B-cells, particularly those in juxtapositionally aposed to T-cells were HLA-DR positive, indicating that these B-cells are probably acting as antigen presenting cells in activating T-cells in situ. Such activated T-cells can produce cytokines which in turn may induce inflammatory reaction in addition to that caused by the accumulated pgl itself.

At first sight our results appear to be in contrast to those of Kobayashi et al (23) it should be noted that we also did not observe positive immunohistological staining (except the background) with any of the other pAbs or mAbs to M.tuberculosis, BCG, M.leprae and M.av., inspite of the fact that these antisera react to cross species antigen. It thus seems that in order to localise the presence of mycobacterial residues in the tissue by immunocytology, specific antibody with high avidity to a particular antigen is needed.

Mycobacterial infection in different individualsmay result in very diverse tissue immune responses, as is well documented in leprosy. Such varying immunoresponses in hosts with different clinical spectrum depend on the type of mycobacterial antigenic epitopes involved. Indeed by immunohistological single and double staining using a panel of mAbs to both cell wall and secretory mycobacterial 30KDa ImCRAC, we could show different types of staining pattern (from weakly diffused or no staining to distinct cellular staining) in the tissues of multibacillary to paucibacillary leprosy patients (33). Interestingly, the distinct cellular staining pattern is observed in the paucibacillary tuberculoid leprosy whereas no staining to weakly diffused staining can be seen in multibacillary lepromatous leprosy.

In the light our present immunohistological data and those of Kobayashi et al strengthen the old testamony of Rubin and Pinnen (39) which reads as follows: "the failure to find mycobacterial bacilli in the tissue is not a convincing argument against mycobacterioses as an etiologic factor, nor are the mycobacterial residues (or occassional bacilli) which are found positive, proof that mycobacterioses is the primary cause for CD".

- **Other Immunological Data**

By applying immunoblotting analysis we could show that IgG antibodies to a 45/48kDa mycobacterial ImCRAC in 65% of CD patients as compared to 20% leprosy, (irrespective of clinical spectrum) 15% in tuberculosis and 20% in other inflammatory bowel diseases (IBD) and <3% in normal healthy controls (40). Encouraged by these findings we extended our serological studies on the measurement of mycobacterial Ab isotypes by both immunoblothing and ELISA using a panel of mycobacterial Im-CRAC purified by SDS-PAGE, (also) subcellular antigenic preparations e.g. P90 (44,45), commercially available A60 (ANDA, Strassbourg, France) different PPD preparations (Straten Serum Laboratories, Denmark) and peptidoglycolipid prepations of M.tuberculosis, M.avium and M.bovis BCG (kind gifts from Dr. A. Kolk, of Laboratory for Tropical Diseases, Amsterdam, The Netherlands), in CD, UC, DC, CC, patients with ankylosing spondylitis (AS) with/without CD, lep, tb and normal individuals.

In immunoblotting most of the individuals including normals, showed varying sero-reactivity to a wide range of mycobacterial antigenic bands. However, 65% of CD patients had significantly increased IgG-Ab to 45/48kDa doublet as compared to 12% of UC and 10% of patients with other IBD. In lep, tb and AS patients and normals the percentanges of sero-reactive individuals were 20, 15, 15 and <5% , respectively.

Particularly the lep and tb patients showed significant sero-reactivities with other mycobacterial ImCRAC e.g. 29/33kDa doublet (for lepromatous lep), 65kDa (for tuberculoid lep) and in the ranges of 58-60kDa, 38-40kDa and 14-22kDa (in case of tb patients). Interestingly, 15% of AS with positive reactivity to 45/48 kDa doublet were also diagnosed as CD patients. Similarly in ELISA, when a cut off value of O.D.405nm of 0.4 at serum dilution of 1:400 was applied, 60% of DC patients had elevated IgGAb to the isolated 45/48kDa doublet. In other IBD patients these Abs were present in 12% UC, <5% DC, 12% AS patients (only with CD) and <3% in normals respectively. IgG Ab to 45/48kDa were also found in 30% of both lep and tb patients. However, additional ELISA Ab isotype measurement to another pannel of mycobacterial ImCRAC e.g.29/33kDa doublet, 65kDa singlet and IgA Ab to P90 in combination with immunoblotting clearly distinguished lep/tb sera from those of CD.

A review of our such differential serological studies has been described in a recent article (44). However, with other mycobacterial antigens we could not find any increased level of antibody titre in CD patients in a disease specific manner; this latter results are compatible with those of Kobayashi et al (26).

These inconsistencies in seroreactivity does not necessarily contradict the hypothesis regarding mycobacterial etiology, since mycobacterial species are so wide spread that all individuals, healthy and diseased, are likely to be sensitised by these organisms and their antigens. Thus universal sero-reactivity of the general population to mycobacterial ImCRAC will be detected, when unpurified antigens or very common antigen such as lipoarabinomannan, or A60 are used; consequently a wide range of overlapping sero-reactivities would likely to be observed.

Therefore, the disagreement about the elevated level of serum antibodies to mycobacteria in CD patients may be due to the failure by previous investigators to identify "disease specific" immunodominant antigens. Our present approach using a pannel of isolated mycobacterial antigens in both immunoblotting and ELISA serology showes that CD patients indeed have raised antibody titre to a particular mycobacterial antigen e.g. 45/48kDa doublet and whereas patients with other inflammatory diseases have antibody titres to other dominant mycobacterial ImCRAC in disease specific manners (41).

In order to substantiate our findings on ELISA serology in CD patients we carried out a longitudinal study. We observed that >180 days after intestinal resection, the mycobacterial Ab to 45/48kDa doublet were reduced by 40% in all (27/17) and below the cut off value in 2 patients. Furthermore there appeared to have a positive correlation between Ab titre and disease activity index (42).

CONCLUDING REMARKS

The present immunohistopathological and serological studies provide evidence for the mycobacterial etiology in the following ways:

1 Immunoenzymatic single and double stainings using a panel of mAbs and pAbs to different bacterial strains with varying specificities show increased acumulation of a specific PGL antigen of M.avium in CD gut tissues as compared to other IBD and normal gut.

2 The m.a.v. PGL-antigen appears to be localised as a boundimmunocomplex in IgA, IgG and IgM positive B-cells. Additionally this mycobacterial degraded product is also found on CD19+ B-cells.

3 This m.a.v. PGL antigen bound B-cells are often HLA-DR positive particularly those juxtapositionally in contact with CD3+-T-cells.

The above mentioned observations raise the questions whether or not the increased accumulation of the m.a.v. pgl-antigen sets the trends of events in sustaining the local activation of T-cells thus causing chronic inflammation of the gut in CD patients. However, transient passage of environmental mycobacteria such as M.avium may not be related to active mycobacterial infections.

4 Additional serological data showed that 65% of CD patients sera have increased IgG Ab 45/48kDa doublet in disease specific manner. Mycobacterial immunity, however, in majority cases is T-cell mediated in respect to bactericidal effect whereas antibody mediated response to mycobacteria has often been related to pathogenesis.

Although the present studies, in no way, provide definitive proof for active mycobacterioses in CD patients, the data indicate that quantative evaluation of m.a.v. pgl-mAb reactive cells in the gut wall of endoscopic material in one hand and ELISA monitoring of patients with 45/48kDa antigen, on the other hand, may be a useful clue for the immunopathology of CD.

ACKNOWLEDGEMENT

The authors acknowledge the support of Subfaculty of Medicine under the project numbers of GNK/DA/004 and GNK/PA/46 to carry-out these studies. Our thanks are also due to Miss Sila Yong for excellent technical assistance and to Drs. H.J.L.G. Blaauwgeers for the initial pathological diagnosis of the patients. We also extend our gratitude to the staff of the Pathology Laboratories for various support in sustaining this investigation.

REFERENCES

1 Thornton J.R., Emmet P.M., Heaton K.W. Diet and Crohn's disease: Characteristics of the pre-illness diet.
Br. Med. J. 2: 762, 1979.

2 Sacher D.B., Auslander M.O., Walfish J.S.: Aetiological theories of inflammatory bowel disease.
Clin. Gastroenterology, 9:231-257, 1980.

3 Krisner J.B., Shorter R.G.: Recent developments in "non-specific" inflammatory bowel disease (Part II),
N. Eng. J. Med., 306: 837-848, 1982.

4 Taub R.N., Schar D., Janowitz H.D. and Siltzbach L.E. Induction of granulomas in mice by inoculation of tissue homogenates from patients with inflammatory bowel disease and sarcoidosis.
Ann. N.Y. Acad. Sci. 278: 560-564, 1976.

5 Mitchell D.N. and Rees R.J.W.. Further observations on the transmissibility of Crohn's disease.
Ann. N.Y. Acad. Sci. 278: 546-549, 1976.

6 Simonowitz D., Block G.E., Ridell R.H., Kraft S.C. and Krisner J.B. The production of an unusual tissue reaction in rabbit bowel injected with Crohn's disease homogenates.
Surgery 82: 211-218, 1977.

7 Cave D.R., Mitchell D.N. and Brooke B.N.: Induction of granulomas in mice by Crohn's disease tissue.
Gastroenterology 75: 632-637, 1978.

8 Ahlberg J., Bergstrand O., Gillstrom P., Holstrom B., Kronevi T. and Reiland S. Negative findings in search for a transmissible agent in Crohn's disease. Acta. Chir.
Scand. Suppl. 482: 45-47, 1978.

9 Thayer W. Executive summary of the A.G.A.- N.F.I.C. sponsored workshop on infectious agents in inflammatory bowel disease.
Dig. Dis. Sci. 24: 781-784, 1979.

10 Dalziel T.K. Chronic interstitial enteritis.
Br. Med. J. 2: 1068-1070.

11 Moschowitz E. and Wilensky A. Non-specific granulomata of the intenstine.
Am. J. Med. Sci. 166: 48-66.

12 Crohn B., Ginzburg L. and Oppenheimer G., Regional iletis, a pathological and clinical entity.
J. Am. Med. Assoc. 99: 1323-1329, 1932.
13 Abrams J.S. and Holder W.D. Tuberculosis of the gastrointestinal tract.
Arch. Surg. (Chicago) 89: 292-293,1964.
14 Wig K.L., Chitkara N.L., Gupta S.P., Kishore K. and Manchada R.L. Ileocecal tuberculosis with particular reference to isolation of Mycobacterium tuberculosis. With a note on its relation to regional ileitis (Crohn's disease). Am. Rev. Respir. Dis. 84: 169-178, 1961.
15 Golde B.W. and McGill C.M.: Aetiology of regional enteritis.
Lancet i: 1144-1145, 1968.
16 Burnham W.R. and Lennard-Jones J.E. Mycobacteria as a possible cause of inflammatory bowel disease.
Lancet ii: 693-696, 1978.
17 Stanford J.L., Dourmashkin R., McIntyre G. and Visuvanathan S. Do mycobacteria exist in alternative physical forms and what part may they play in the aetiology in inflammatory bowel disease, p. 503-508; In R.P. MacDermott (ed.) Inflammatory bowel disease.
Current status and future approach. Elsevier Science Publishing Inc. Amsterdam, 1988.
18 Chiodini R.J., Van Kruiningen H.J., Merkal R.S., Thayer W.R. and Coutu J.A.: Characteristics of an unclassified Mycobacterium species isolated from patients with Crohn's disease.
J. Clin. Microbiol. 20: 966-971, 1984.
19 Chiodini R.J., Van Kruiningen H.J., Thayer W.R., Merkal R.S., Coutu J.A.: The possible role of mycobacteria in inflammatory bowel disease I.
Dig. Dis. Sci. 29: 1073-1079, 1984.
20 Blaauwgeers H.J.L.G., Mulder C.J.J., Das P.K., Haagsma J. and Tytgat G.N.J.: Crohn's disease, a mycobacterial aetiology?
Eur. J. Gastroenterol. Hepatol. 2: 237-240,1990.
21 Haga Y: Mycobacteria in Crohn's disease (in Japanese).
Jpn. J. Gastroenterol. 23: 2325-2333, 1986.
22 Van Kruiningen H.J., Thayer W.R., Chiodini R.J., Meuton D.J. and Coutu J.A.: An immunoperoxidase search for mycobacteria in Crohn's disease; p. 547-552.
In R.P. MacDermott (ed.), Inflammatory Bowel Disease.
Current status and future approach. Elsevier Science Publishing Inc. Amsterdam.
23 Kobayashi K., Blaser M.J. and Brown W.R.: Immunohistochemical examination for mycobacteria in intestinal tissues from patients with Crohn's disease.
Gastroenterol. 96: 1009-1115, 1989.
24 Jiwa N.M., Mulder C.J.J., Van den Berg F.M., Tytgat G.N.J., Haagsma J. and Walboomers J.M.M. Elevated IgG to mycobacterial PPD's in Crohn's disease. Inflammatory bowel disease: current status and future approach eds. by MacDermott R.P., Amsterdam: Elsevier Publishing Inc., p. 543-546, 1988.

25 Cho S.N., Brennan P.J., Yoshimura H.H., Korelitz B.I. and Graham D.Y. Mycobacterial aetiology of Crohn's disease: Serologic study using common mycobacterial antigens and a species specific glycolipid antigen from Mycobacterium paratuberculosis.
GUT 27: 1353-1356, 1986.

26 Kobayashi K., Brown W.R., Brennan P.J. and Blaser M.J.: Serum antibodies to mycobacterial antigens in active Crohn's disease.
Gastroenterol. 94: 1404-1411, 1988.

27 Cohen I.R. and Yong D.B.: Autoimmmunity, microbial immunity and immunological homunculus.
Immunology today 12: 105-110, 1991.

28 Rook G.A.W. and Stanford J.L.: Slow bacterial infections or autoimmunity.
Immunology today in press, 1992.

29 Rook G.A.W. An integrated view of the immunology of mycobacterioses in guineapigs, mice and men. In Ratledge C., Stanford J.L. eds. The Biology of the Mycobacteria Vol.2, London, New York: Academic Press, p. 279-319, 1983.

30 Das P.K., Haque A. and Bos J.D.: SIS in relation to bacterial and parasite infection. In Bos J.D. ed. Skin Immune System (SIS), Boca Raton U.S.A.: CRC press, p. 403-446, 1990.

31 Radema S.A., Hommes D.W., Fockens P., Stronkhorst A., Jansen J., Zhao Y., Tytgat G.N.J. and Van Deventer S.J.H.: Cytokine Induction in experimental and ulcerative colitis, in press.

32 Van der Loos C.J.M., Das P.K., Van den Oord J.J. and Houthoff H.J.: Multiple immunoenzyme staining techniques. Use of fluorescinated, biotynalated and unlabelled monoclonal antibodies.
J. Immunol. Methods 1117: 45-52,1989.

33 Rambukkana A., Das P.K., Krieg S. and Faber W.R.: Association of mycobacterial 30 KDa region proteins with cutaneous infiltrates of leprosy lesions: Evidence for the involvement of the major mycobacterial secreted proteins in local immune response of leprosy; Scand. J. Immunol., in press 1992.

34 Das P.K., Rambukkana A., Baas J.G., Groothuis D.G. and Halperin M.: Enzymelinked immunosorbent assay for distinguishing serological response of lepromatous and tuberculoid leprosies to the 29/33 KDa and 64 KDa antigens of mycobacterium tuberculosis.
J. Clin. Microbiol. 28: 379-382, 1990.

35 Rambukkana A., Das P.K., Chand A., Baas J.G., Groothuis D.G. and Kolk A.H.G.: Subcellular distribution of monoclonal antibody defined epitopes on Mycobacterium tuberculosis proteins in the 30 KDa region: Identification and localisation of 29/33 KDa doublet proteins on mycobacterial cell wall.
Scand. J. Immunol. 33: 763-775, 1991.

36 Kolk A.H.J., Evers R., Groothuis D.G., Gillis H. and Kuijper S. Production and characterisation of monoclonal antibodies against specific serotypes of Mycobacterium avium and the Mycobacterium avium - Mycobacterium intracellulaire - Mycobacterium scrofulaceum complex.
Infect. Immun. 57: 2514-2521, 1989.

37 Das P.K., Blaauwgeers H.J.L.G., Slob A.W., Spies J., Chaud A. and Houthoff H.J. On the mycobacterial aetiology of Crohn's disease: relevant immunological studies.
Gastroenterology 94: A88, 1988.

38 Das P.K., Stronkhorst A., Blaauwgeers H.J.L.G., Slob A.W. and Tytgat G.N.J.: "Is Crohn's disease a mycobacterial disease ?" Immunohistological evidence.
Gastroenterology, in press, 1992.

39 Rubin E.H. and Pinner M. Sarcoidosis: one case report and literature review of autopsied cases.
Am. Rev. Tuberc. 49: 146-149, 1944.

40 Das P.K., Blaauwgeers H.J.L.G., Slob A.W., Yong S.L. and Rambukkana A. Mycobacterial antibody (Myc Ab) response in relation to Crohn's disease (CD): Gastroenterology 96: A111, 1989.

41 Das P.K. and Grange J.M.: Review: Mycobacteria in relation to tissue immune response and pathogenesis; Med. Microbiol., in press, 1992.

42 Kreuzpaintner G., Das P.K., Blaauwgeers H.J.L.G., Köble R., Slob A.W., Wallner A., Strohmeyer G.: Der Einfluss der Resektion erkrankter Dermabschnitte auf spezifische mykobakterielle Antikörper bei Patienten mit Morbus Crohn. Zeitschrift für Gastroenterologie (German J. Gastroenterol.) B662E, p. 497, A102, 1990.

MYCOBACTERIUM PARATUBERCULOSIS AND CROHN'S DISEASE

J.D.Sanderson, M.T.Moss, M.L.V.Tizard &
J. Hermon-Taylor

Department of Surgery, St.George's Hospital Medical School,
Cranmer Terrace, London, SW17 ORE. U.K.

Mycobacterium paratuberculosis has been grown in bacillary form in in-vitro culture and identified by conventional means in a very small proportion of Crohn's disease patients [1-4]. Other studies have shown that this organism contains multiple copies of a DNA insertion element IS900, stably integrated in its genome [5,6]. IS900 provides a convenient target for the sensitive and specific detection of M.paratuberculosis by polymerase chain reaction (PCR) [7,8].

Full thickness samples of intestinal tissue were obtained immediately after surgical resection from 40 patients with Crohn's disease, 23 patients with ulcerative colitis and 40 control patients without IBD (colon cancer 35, gastric ulcer 2, sigmoid diverticulitis 2, small gut sarcoma 1). Tissues samples were chopped, homogenised and centrifuged to decrease proportionately the amount of human DNA in the final extract by pelletting some host nuclei. DNA was prepared using enzymic digestion and cycles of phenol/chloroform extraction. Oligonucleotide PCR primers were selected to amplify a 400bp portion of the 5' region of IS900. Primers were selected on the basis of minimum 3' base mis-match, freedom from involvement in IS900 secondary structure and specificity in relation to the known DNA sequences of other insertion elements in this family [9-12]. PCR conditions were optimised and reactions carried out in triplicate using 5μl aliquots of tissue DNA extract. Each triplicate assay was accompanied by a simultaneous no-template PCR control. Throughout the study, scrupulous precautions were taken to exclude artefact due to laboratory contamination.

Of the 40 non-IBD controls 5 (12.5%) were positive for M.paratuberculosis. All these were samples of apparently normal colon from patients having operations for colon cancer. 1 of 23 (4.3%) ulcerative colitis tissues was positive. Of the 40 Crohn's disease samples, 26

(65%) were positive for M.paratuberculosis in samples from both diseased small intestine and colon. All PCR controls were negative.

These findings show that there is a previously unsuspected colonic prevalence of M.paratuberculosis in non-IBD people in southern England. If the experimentally unequivocal presence of M.paratuberculosis in the diseased tissues of a substantial majority of patients with Crohn's disease was an opportunistic invasion, we could reasonably expect to find a broadly similar situation in ulcerative colitis. The low figure for ulcerative colitis favours an aetiological relationship between M.paratuberculosis and a proportion of Crohn's disease.

A tissue microbial abundance below the limit of detection by our present methods (about 300 M.paratuberculosis genomes per gram of tissue) may account for some of the PCR negative results on Crohn's disease patients in the present study. An additional and equally probable explanation would be the involvement of another mycobacterium very closely related to M.paratuberculosis and also specifically capable of causing chronic enteritis in an appropriately susceptible host.

Mycobacterium paratuberculosis is a known specific cause of chronic enteritis with a varying clinico-pathological picture and ease of identification by culture in cattle, sheep, goats, pigs, dogs, horses, chickens, rabbits and primates [13-16]. It is probably the cause of a significant proportion of the chronic enteritis, Crohn's disease, in humans as well.

REFERENCES

1 Chiodini RJ, Van Kruiningen HJ, Merkal RS, Thayer WR, Coutu JA. Characteristics of an unclassified mycobacterium species isolated from patients with Crohn's disease. J Clin Microbiol. 1984; 20: 966-971.

2 Haagsma J, Mulder CJJ, Eger A, Bruins J, Ketel RJ & Tytgat GNJ. Mycobacterium species isolated from patients with Crohn's disease. In MacDermott RP (ed.) Inflammatory Bowel Disease: Current Status and Future Approach. Amsterdam: Excerpta Medica. 1988; 535-7.

3 Coloe P, Wilks CR, Lightfoot D, Tosolini FA. Isolation of Mycobacterium paratuberculosis in Crohn's Disease. Austral Microbiol. 1986; 7:188A.

4 Gitnick G, Collins J, Beaman B, Brooks D, Arthur M, Imaeda T & Palieschesky M. Preliminary Report on Isolation of Mycobacteria from Patients with Crohn's Disease. Dig Dis & Sci. 1989; 34: 925-932.

5 McFadden JJ, Thompson J, Hull E, Hampson S, Stanford J & Hermon-Taylor J. The use of cloned DNA probes to examine organisms isolated from Crohn's disease tissue. In MacDermott RP (ed.) Inflammatory Bowel Disease: Current Status and Future Approach, Amsterdam: Excerpta Medica.1988: 515-520.

6 Green EP, Tizard MLV, Moss MT, Thompson J, Winterbourne DJ, McFadden JJ & Hermon-Taylor J. Sequence and characteristics of IS900, an insertion element identified in human Crohn's Disease isolate of Mycobacterium paratuberculosis. Nuc Acid Res. 1989; 17: 9063-73.
7 Moss MT, Green EP, Tizard MLV, Malik Z & Hermon-Taylor J Specific detection of Mycobacterium paratuberculosis by DNA hybridisation with a fragment of the insertion element IS900. Gut. 1991; 32: 395-398.
8 Vary PH, Anderson PR, Green E, Hermon-Taylor J & McFadden JJ. Use of highly specific DNA probes and the polymerase chain reaction to detect mycobacterium paratuberculosis in Johne's disease. J Clin Microbiol. 1990; 28: 933-937.
9 Moss MT, Malik Z, Tizard MLV, Green EP, Sanderson JD & Hermon-Taylor J. IS902, an insertion element of the chronic enteritis causing Mycobacterium avium subsp.silvaticum. J Gen Microbiol. 1992; 138: 139-145.
10 Bruton CJ & Chater KF. Nucleotide sequence of IS110, an insertion sequence of Streptomyces coelicolor A3(2). Nuc Acid Res. 1987; 15: 7053-7065.
11 Leskiw BK, Mevarech M, Barritt LS, Jensen SE, Henderson DJ, Hopwood DA, Bruton CJ & Chater KF. Discovery of an insertion sequence, IS116, from Streptomyces clavuligerus and its relatedness to other transposable elements from actinomycetes. J Gen Microbiol. 1990; 136: 1251-1258.
12 Ashby MK & Bergquist PL. Cloning and Sequence of IS1000, a Putative Insertion Sequence from Thermus thermophilus HB8. Plasmid. 1990; 24: 1-11.
13 Chiodini RJ, van Kruiningen HJ & Merkal RS. Ruminant paratuberculosis (Johne's disease): the current status and future prospects. Cornell Vet. 1984; 74: 218-262.
14 Stamp JT & Watt JA. Johne's Disease in Sheep. J.Comp.Path. 1954; 64: 26-40.
15 Mokresh AH, Czuprynski CJ & Butler DG. A Rabbit Model for Study of Mycobacterium paratuberculosis Infection. Inf. Imm. 1989; 57: 3798-3807.
16 McClure HM, Chiodini RJ, Anderson DC, Swenson RB, Thayer WR & Coutu JA. Mycobacterium paratuberculosis (Johne's disease) in a colony of stump-tail macaques (Macaca arctoides). J Inf Dis. 1987; 155: 1011-1019.

RABBITS AND SEVERE COMBINED IMMUNODEFICIENT (SCID) MICE AS ANIMAL MODELS FOR MYCOBACTERIA IN CROHN'S DISEASE.

D.G. Butler, DVM, PhD,

Department of Clinical Studies, Ontario Veterinary College, University of Guelph, Canada

This research reflects my clinical interests as a large animal veterinarian in a disease of cattle and small ruminants called Paratuberculosis or Johne's Disease (1,2) and my research interests in comparative gastroenterology specifically, infectious gastroentitis. Mycobacterium paratuberculosis (MPTB), the cause of Johne's Disease inhabits the intestinal mucosa of the ileal and cecal area and adjacent lymph nodes, causing a chronic granulomatous enteritis. The organism is transmitted horizontally by the ingestion of food and water contaminated with feces from an infected animal shedding the organism (3). Resistance to infection increases with age (4) and depending on the number of exposures and the dose of organisms per exposure, the status of natural resistance and the active immune response to the challenge, one of two outcomes is possible. Either the animal may eliminate the organism or much less commonly a persistent infection is established (5). In the latter instance, following an incubation period of one or more years during which there may or may not be an immune response and fecal shedding of the organism, clinical disease becomes evident. Terminally, emaciation occurs with or without diarrhea (2).

The long incubation period and low frequency of clinical disease following natural and experimental infection of large domestic animals and the high costs of purchase and maintenance of these animals prompted our use of the neonatal rabbit as an animal model to study the pathogenesis and pathophysiology of MPTB. Much of this work has previously been reported (6, 7). In the interest of summarizing the usefulness or applicability of the rabbit as an animal model for the study of mycobacteria in Crohn's Disease, I will briefly summarize some additional research done by Dr. A. H. Mokresh when he was a graduate student in my laboratory at the University of Wisconsin. I want to also acknowledge the contribution to this work of another graduate student, Dr. J.Bell and several colleagues at the University of Wisconsin, C. Czprynski, PhD, D. Manning, PhD, A. Kiorpes, DVM, PhD and C. Luker, BS.

Pregnant, pasteurella- and coccidia-free New Zealand White rabbits were purchased one to two weeks before parturition, housed in separate cages in an isolation room and allowed to kindle naturally. Following parturition, one dow and litter were designated as controls and moved to a separate isolation room and the remaining does and their offspring were assigned to the test group. On days 1 and 2 after birth, each neonate was inoculated orally by gavage with a total volume of 2 ml containing 3.6 X 10^8 CFU of M.paratuberculosis ATCC 19698 (n=15) or 2 ml containing 2.6 X 10^8 CFU of M.paratuberculosis 22206 (n=3) a field isolate of bovine origin obtained from the Wisconsin Central Animal Health Laboratory. To avoid cannibalism by the does, plastic disposable gloves were worn and the newborns were dusted with talcum powder each time they were handled. The rabbits were weaned at 7 weeks, observed daily, weighed weekly and necropsied at 9 months of age. No cannibalism occurred. No respiratory problems were observed in the does or offspring at any time during the experiment. This was attributed to the pasteurella-free status of the does, the effectiveness of the protocol for handling the neonates and the clean environment in which they were raised. Further, we concluded that the supposed predilection of neonatal rabbits to develop respiratory disease when stressed by handling and repeated manipulation was very much over emphasized particularly if pasteurella-induced respiratory disease was prevented.

Although intermittent diarrhea starting after 4 months of age was observed in 9 out of 13 rabbits (69%) inoculated with MPTB 19698, and 3 out of the 3 inoculated with MPTB 22206 when necropsied at 9 months after infection, gross lesions were not seen in any rabbits. Further, only 3 out of 13 rabbits given the MPTB 19698 and 0 of 3 given MPTB 22206 had histological evidence of intestinal granulomas. MPTB was not cultured from any of the feces or intestinal tissue homogenates collected at necropsy after 3 months of incubation. However, after 11 - 15 months of continuous incubation, bacterial colonies were observed growing on the Herrold's egg yolk agar medium (HEYM) supplemented with mycobactin J. but not on comparably inoculated HEYM without mycobactin J.
from 8 of the 16 MPTB inoculated rabbits. Negative cultures from infected and control rabbits incubated a further 9 months (24 months in total) did not show any bacterial growth.

In addition to being mycobactin dependent, the slow growing colonies isolated on the HEYM were 0.5 mm in diameter, translucent, with a tendency to grow down into the agar and did not take up an acid-fast stain. Colonies excised from the agar and processed for transmission electronmicroscopy revealed cell wall-deficient organisms consisting of pleomorphic, electron-dense, round to elongated bodies. The electron-dense bodies were composed of granular structures enclosed by a poorly defined plasma membrane with multiple outer projections. These organisms lacked the usual outer triple cell wall layer associated with mycobacteria and appeared to be cell wall-deficient forms of mycobacterium spp. similar to those first isolated from patients with colitis by Burnham et. at. in 1978 (8) and by Chiodini et. at. in 1986 (9) from patients with Crohn's Disease.

Because of the small quantity of the cell wall-deficient colonies and the lack of specificity of the available probe, attempts to do a genomic DNA extraction and hybridization to confirm that the slow-growing wall-deficient form was MPTB were unsuccessful. However, given its mycobactin J. dependence and that the colonies only grew from tissues and feces collected from MPTB infected animals, we feel the isolate was a transformed MPTB organism. Whether that transformation took place in the rabbit or whether it occurred during the decontamination procedure using 0.75% Hexadecyl Cetylpyridinium Chloride (HPC) could not be established. Likewise, the relationship of these cell wall-deficient organisms to inflammatory bowel disease remains an open question.

Once I moved from the University of Wisconsin to the University of Guelph, in Ontario Canada, I no longer had access to pasteurella-free rabbits without importing them, and that proved prohibitively expensive. Fortunately, I was able to initiate experiments using severe combined immunodeficient (SCID) mice kindly provided by Dr. Anne Croy, a colleague in the Department of Biomedical Sciences at the University of Guelph. Because SCID/bg mutant mice lack functional T- and B-cells and have reduced NK activity (10), it seemed reasonable to expect that these mice might be very susceptible to infection with MPTB. The research I will share now in an attempt to indicate the potential usefulness and applicability of the SCID/bg mouse as an animal model for the study of mycobacterium in Crohn's Disease has primarily been conducted by Dr. George Mutwiri DVM, a doctoral student and Dr. Olimpo Oliver, DVM, MS, another graduate student in my laboratory. Several technical staff including A. Bashiri, DVM, J. Greenwood, N. Von Althen, and A. Hathway and several colleagues at the University of Guelph (A. Croy, DVM, PhD, S. Rosendal, DVM, PhD, and M. Ruka, DVM, PhD, and R. Duncan, DVM, PhD., at the Animal Disease Research Institute (ADRI) in Ottawa has also contributed to this research.

Six to eight week old Scid/Scid.bg/bg mutants of CB17/C57BL mice of mixed sexes were held in microisolator cages with filter caps and fed sterile food and water. Because of our experience with the bovine field isolate in the rabbit studies, we decided to use a bovine isolate of MPTB extracted from frozen bovine intestine provided by Dr. Robert Duncan, a colleague studying Johne's Disease at the ADRI. Scraped intestinal mucosa was homogenized in 0.75% HPC (1:35) left for 18 hours at room temperature and then pelleted by centrifugation and washed repeatedly and suspended in sterile pyrogen-free saline. Autoclaved test inoculum to kill the MPTB was used as the control inoculum for all the experiments. Test and control inocula were stored at -70°C, thawed and warmed to body temperature and diluted 1:3 with sterile pyrogen-free saline before use. Test mice each received one dose ($1\text{-}2 \times 10^5$) of MPTB intraperitoneally at 6-8 weeks of age. Controls received a comparable inoculum autoclaved to kill the MPTB or sterile pyrogen-free saline.

Test and control mice were anesthetized at 2, 3, 4, 6, 8, 12, 16, 22 and 26 weeks post-infection and bled. The peritoneal cavity was lavaged with 1 ml of sterile pyrogen-free saline and the mice were then killed. Samples from all vital organs were collected for histology.

Clinically by 4 months post-infection, test mice were smaller in size and looked clinically ill with rough hair coats and a tendency to huddle together much of the time. In fact, starting 12 weeks post-infection, test mice weighed significantly less than control but appeared to maintain their appetites and had no clinical evidence of diarrhea. By 26 weeks post-infection, the test mice at necropsy had very dry emaciated looking carcasses lacking fat. The livers were pale and mottled, the spleen were extremely enlarged. Histologically, acid-fast bacteria were first observed in the gut at 12 weeks post-infection in the submucosa of the villi, associated with many mononuclear cells and relatively few PMN's. By 26 weeks post-infection the number of organisms had increased tremendously. Interestingly, large numbers of acid-fast bacteria were present in peritoneal macrophages obtained by lavage of the abdomen at all time periods up to 26 weeks when the experiment was terminated. Histologically up to 3 weeks post-infection isolated aggregates of both mononuclear and PMN cells were seen with 1-2 acid-fast bacteria only in the liver. Between 4-8 weeks post-infection distinct focal lesions comprised of mononuclear and PMN cells in equal numbers with the occasional giant cell and increasing numbers of acid-fast bacilli were observed. Between 12-26 weeks, lesions in the liver coalesced, developed collagen deposits and became predominantly epithelioid/mononuclear in nature with very few PMN's and increasing numbers of acid-fast organisms stuffed within what appeared to be macrophages. MPTB was cultured only from the test inoculum and liver, spleen and gut of test mice using HEYM with mycobactin J. No growth was obtained from the control inoculum or control mice. TNF1-α assays on plasma from test and control mice were negative as were all samples of plasma tested for murine immunoglobins. To date, we have concluded that MPTB infection can be readily established in Scid/bg mice with a single intraperitoneal injection of $1\text{-}2 \times 10^5$ organisms; that acid-fast organisms persist in the peritoneal macrophages obtained by abdominal lavage without gross or cytologic evidence of peritonitis: and that test mice become progressively more emaciated with time while apparently retaining an adequate feed intake. This cachexia does not seem to require competent lymphocytes and TNF-α. Finally, the lesions developed in a time dependent fashion first appearing in the liver, then the spleen and finally the gut. The lesions which consisted mainly of macrophages with intracellular acid-fast organisms in ever increasing numbers, involved relatively few PMN cells.

We see this model of potential use for the study of immunopathogenesis cachexia and therapy of MPTB diseases of man and animals. Also, it may be of use to facilitate the isolation of slow-growing difficult or non-cultivable Mycobacterium from clinical specimens.

REFERENCES

1 Johne, H.A., and L. Frothingham. 1895. Ein eigentumlicher Fall Vontuberkulose beim Rind. Dtsch. Ztschr. Tiermed. Path. 21:438-454.

2 Chiodini, R.J., H.J. Van Kruingen, and R.S. Merkal. 1984. Ruminant paratuberculosis (Johne's Disease): The current status and future prospects. Cornell Vet. 74:218-262.

3 Thomas, G.W., 1985. Johne's Disease (paratuberculosis) in goats. Veterinary Annual. Editors, C.S.G. Gruncell, F.W.G. Hill, M.Z. Raw. Bristol: Scientechnica. 25:231-235.

4 Hagan, W.A. 1938. Age as a factor in susceptibility to Johne's disease. Cornell Vet. 38:34-40.

5 Payne, J.M. and J.D. Rankin. 1961. The pathogenesis of experimental Johne's disease in calves. Res. Vet. Sci. 2:167-174.

6 Mokresh, A.H., C.J. Czuprynski and D.G. Butler. 1989. Rabbit Model for study of Mycobacterium paratuberculosis infection. Infect. Immun. 57:3798-3807.

7 Mokresh, A.H., and D.G. Butler. (1990). Granulomatous Enteritis following oral inoculation of newborn rabbits with Mycobacterium paratuberculosis of bovine origin. Can. J.Vet.Res. 54:313-319.

8 Burnham, W.R., and J.E. Lennard-Jones. 1978. Mycobacteria as a possible cause of inflammatory bowel disease. Lancet. 9:693-696.

9 Chiodini, R.J., H.J.Van Kruiningen, W.R. Thayer, and J.A. Coutu. 1986. Spheroplastic phase of Mycobacteria isolated from patients with Crohn's disease. J.Clin.Microbiol. 24:357-363.

10 Croy, B.A., and C. Chapeau. 1990. Evaluation of the pregnancy immunotropism hypothesis by assessment of the reproductive performance of young adult mice of genotype scid/scid.bg/bg. J.Reprod.Fert. 88:231-239.

IMMUNOTHERAPEUTICAL APPROACHES TO CROHN'S DISEASE IN VIEW OF A POSSIBLE PATHOGENIC ROLE OF MYCOBACTERIAL ANTIGENS.

Arnold Stronkhorst, Guido N.J. Tytgat, Sander J.H. van Deventer.

Dept. Gastroenterology, Academic Medical Center, Meibergdreef 9, 1105 AZ, Amsterdam, The Netherlands

INTRODUCTION

The immune system of the intestinal tract has been extensively studied. The lamina propria of adults is heavy populated with a variety of lymphoid cells: B- and T-lymphocytes, plasma cells, macrophages, mast cells, eosinophils and basophils. In normal subjects the majority of the B-cells are committed to IgA synthesis (90%), the residual 10% being represented (in order of decreasing frequency) by IgM, IgG, IgE and IgD producing plasma cells. These cells, which are located diffusely in the mucosa and more organized in Peyer's patches, together with the an intact mucosal layer provide an effective barrier to the antigenic food load, that passes the bowel daily. Small amounts of antigen can transmigrate through the mucosa either by endo/pinocytic processes or via the tight junction complex. The production of antibodies to antigens penetrating the barrier is a physiological process that usually results in systemic tolerance. Changes in these immunological processes, caused by an altered mucosal barrier, an abnormal antigen-antibody or antigen-antigen presenting cell response, may play a role in the pathogenesis of Crohn's disease.

Although many immunological changes have been documented in Crohn's disease, it still is not clear whether these changes are a primary disorder of the immune system or secondary to the inflammatory process; in both cases the initiating process or agent that leads to inflammation remains unknown. In this chapter we will discuss some immunological changes that can be observed in Crohn's disease patients. We will speculate on the pathogenic role of mycobacterial antigens and suggest a novel immuno therapeutical intervention strategy.

ANTIGEN PRESENTATION AND T-CELL ACTIVATION IN CROHN'S DISEASE

In Crohn's disease an increased permeability of the intestinal mucosa for larger molecules may exist[1,2], probably due to an abnormal tight junction structure[3]. Various (food derived-?) antigens can pass the mucosal layer by pino- or endocytosis, but oral and systemic tolerance for most of them is derived early in live by respectively mucosal IgA production and specific non-responsiveness of the systemic immune system to luminal antigens. It is not clear whether the permeability for very large molecular structures such as mycobacteria or mycobacterial antigens is increased in Crohn's disease. Besides a primary change in permeability it is also possible that penetration of antigens in the inflamed mucosa is a secondary process which perpetuates a destructive primary immune response. The supposed primary increased permeability is not obligate for immune activation, because enterocytes may exhibit antigen presenting capacities, shown by there expression of HLA-DR[4,5,6].

The importance of T-lymphocytes within the normal gut and gut-associated lymphoid tissue is generally accepted: their precise role, however, is uncertain. In the lamina propria most T-lymphocytes express the CD4 (helper) phenotype, whereas in the epithelal layer the CD8 (cytotoxic / suppressor) subtype dominates. The CD4+ cells are predominantly of the helper-inducer and cytolytic subtype, and less frequently of the suppressor-inducer phenotypes[7]. In Crohn's disease there is an influx of inflammatory cells into the diseased area and local production of soluble mediators of inflammation has been shown[8,9]. The pivotal role of T-cells in Crohn's disease is well known[10]. There is an increased number of mucosal T-cells, but the CD4 to CD8 ratio is the same as in control subjects[11]. Earlier immuno-histopathological reports could not show an increase in T-cell activation markers[12,13]. This in contrast to the fact that mononuclear cells isolated from mucosa from Crohn's disease patients did show a slight increase in the expression of these markers[14]. Later studies showed that activated T-cells are abundantly present the submucosa of children with Crohn's disease, in contrast to mucosa of ulcerative colitis patients[15,16]. T-cell activation is not only evident in histological specimens[17,18] but can also be shown in peripheral blood: even the serum level of soluble inter-leukin-2 receptor is increased[19,20]. The total numbers of CD4 and CD8 positive lymphocytes in peripheral blood of Crohn's disease patients are normal, but the T-cells are activated as they express CD25 (interleukin-2 receptor) on their surface[21].

In case of HLA class II restricted antigen presentation, as in type IV immune response, an antigen (fig. 1) is processed by the antigen presenting cell (enterocyte, mononuclear cell, dendritic cell) and presented on its surface by a MHC class II molecule. This complex is

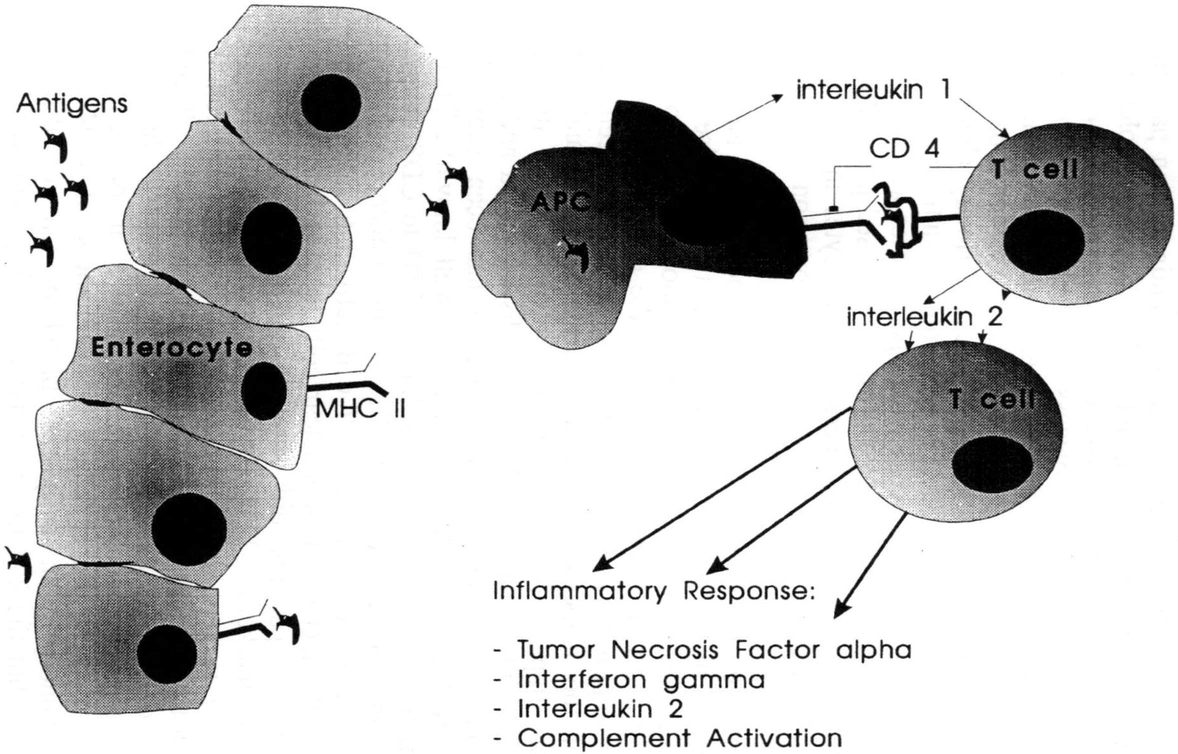

The antigens on the luminal side of the mucosa transmigrate through the epithelial layer, either by endo-/pinocytosis or by the tight junction complex. In case of HLA-restricted antigen presentation as in Crohn's disease the antigen is processed by the antigen presenting cell (APC) and presented on its surface by the class II major histocompatibility complex (MHC II). The antigen presenting cell can either be an enterocyte, monocyte/ macrophage or dendritic cell. The MHC II-antigen complex is recognized by the T-cell receptor. Additional binding by the CD4 molecule (integrin) and a costimulatory signal are necessary for T-cell activation. This in turn leads to the inflammatory response.

recognized by the T helper 1 (Th1) cell receptor. Th1 cells mediate delayed type hypersensitivity[22]. Additional bindings (integrins) and a costimilatory signal (interleukin-1) are necessary for T-cell activation[23]. The antigen(s) to which those T-cells react are still unknown. There identification however would be a major step forward in our understanding of Crohn's disease. Mycobacteria elicit a cellular immune response in their hosts. This response usually leads to protective immunity, but may sometimes be accompanied by immunopathology due to delayed type hypersensitivity (like in tuberculoid leprosy). Mycobacterial antigens are capable of creating a granulomatous inflammation[24], in which mononuclear cells play an important role. Living mycobacteria are not necessary in this proces. Mycobacterial antigens can be shown in mucosa of Crohn's disease patients[25] and Thayer showed that serum antibodies to mycobacterial antigens are more often present in Crohn's disease patients[26]. Mycobacteria selectively induce human T-cells with a Th1-like cytokine profile[27]. Lymphocytes from Crohn's disease patients show marked suppressor activity when stimulated with M.paratuberculosis[28]. These immunological findings may explain why Crohn's disease is a transmural inflammation: the mycobacterial antigen is passing through the mucosa one way or another and subsequently processed by the antigen presenting cell (APC). Then in the lamina propria the T-cell receptor of the T-helper (CD4 +) cell recognizes the antigen-MHC II complex. This results in T-cell activation and a granulomatous transmural inflammation moderated by tumor necrosis factor α, τ interferon, and interleukin-2. Its however not clear what causes the perpetuating immune response and subsequent inflammation.

IMMUNOTHERAPY

The ideal immunosuppressive therapy would be either to neutralize the causative antigen, or to delete all reactive T-cell clones, without affecting the normal immune response. Somewhat less specifically, one could interfere with the antigen presenting process. As can be seen in figure 1. intervening in the antigen presenting pathway provides opportunities for immunotherapy. Because the antigen which causes the immune response in Crohn's disease is still unknown, no vaccination, antibodies or desensibilisation are available.

As T-cells play a central role in all immune responses, they are a primary target for any immuno-therapeutic intervention strategy. For many years polyclonal antibodies that suppress T-cell functions have been investigated as immunosuppressive agents in a variety of diseases. With the development of monoclonal antibodies, specific immunotherapy directed against T-cells became available and had promising results in both animal models and (auto-)immune diseases[29,30]. Monoclonal antibody treatment has largely been applied clinically in cancer and modulation of the immune response to produce immunosuppression for treatment of autoimmune and graft versus host diseases. It is also very effective in the treatment of acute allograft rejection[31]. Human monoclonal antibodies have been used in both viral and bacterial infections[32]. Some monoclonal antibodies are now registered for clinical use, for example OKT3 in allograft rejection. Problems with monoclonal antibody therapy were recognized soon, because anti-(murine-) antibody production limited therapeutic possibilities[33]. Furthermore there are many side effects in murine- and non specific (for example OKT3-) monoclonal antibody therapy. New "humanized" chimeric and recombinant monoclonal antibodies have promising therapeutic prospects. Interference with in the antigen presentation by blocking the T-cell receptor, the CD4 receptor, the interleukin-1ß pathway or the interleukin-2 receptor all are therapeutical options. Other , less specific, strategies consist of blockade of the inflammatory response by antibodies directed against tumor necrosis factor-α, interleukin-2, interferon-τ or their receptors. Currently some of these monoclonal antibody therapies are tested in clinical trials.

The treatment of Crohn's disease with Corticosteroids, Azathioprine / 6-mercaptopurine[34], and 5-Aminosalicylic acid is well accepted and needs no further discussion in this chapter.

Cyclosporine is a novel immunosuppressant, widely used in organ transplantation, that has a selective effect on T-cell mediated immune responses[35]. Cyclosporine is able to reduce expression of Class II molecules on the epithelium in a dramatic way. It also reduces IL-2 and hence τ-interferon production. Cyclosporine has proven to have a beneficial effect in active chronic Crohn's disease patients who were resistant to or intolerant of corticosteroids[36]. Cyclosporine therapy during three month was well tolerated and no serious adverse events were observed, but is associated with a risk of nephropathy.

- **Anti CD4 antibody treatment**

Anti-CD4 treatment in Crohn's disease seems rational in review of the antigen presenting pathway and T-cell activation in Crohn's disease, as described above. Depletion of CD4+ cells is correlated with rapid improvement in an prototypic model of T-cell-mediated autoimmunity: experimental allergic encephalomyelitis[37]. Reports of remissions of Crohn's disease in patients infected with the HIV virus provide additional arguments for anti-CD4 treatment in Crohn's disease[38]. In these cases remission of Crohn's disease occurred simultaneously with a decrease in CD4 cells. In phase I trials, rheumatoid arthritis, which is also characterized by a granulomatous inflammation and T-cell activation, responds to the treatment with murine monoclonal antibodies against the CD4+ (T helper) cells[39,40]. The effect on remission of symptoms after one week of therapy lasted 3 weeks to more then 5 months. Only short-lasting low grade fever on the first day of treatment was seen. However in six out of eight patients an anti-mouse-Ig response developed. This can cause problems (ineffectiveness, allergic response) in longterm treatment of these chronic diseased patients. Currently we are evaluating a chimeric (mouse / human) anti-CD4 monoclonal antibody in Crohn's disease patients, with promising results and without serious side effects. These antibodies have a human IgG constant part and a mouse anti-CD4 variable part. We assume that humanizing the antibody causes less antigenetic response and a longer half live.

- **Anti TNFα treatment**

Both mycobacterial and Crohn's disease are characterized by a granulomatous, transmural inflammation of the bowel. Tumor necrosis factor alpha (TNFα) plays a very important and perhaps pivotal role in granulomatous diseases[41,42,43]. Blocking TNFα prevents the formation of granuloma's[44]. TNFα is in increased amounts present in mucosa and stool of patients with active IBD[45,46]. TNFα can be controlled by reducing its production, TNF-neutralizing antibodies or by blocking the TNF-receptor. Several studies, using murine or murine/human chimeric antibodies, have been initiated in septicemia, and the results from a phase I study have been published[47]. To our knoledge, anti-TNF therapy has not been investigated in Crohn's disease.

Pentoxifylline (a xanthine derivative) has been described to counteract endotoxin induced effects in different animal models[48,49]. Pentoxifylline inhibits in macrophage cultures the synthesis of mRNA for TNFα[50] and therefore is an alternative for anti-TNF antibody therapy. Pentoxifylline is also able to inhibit the inflammatory action of interleukin-1 and TNFα on neutrophil function[51]. No data are available on the effect of pentoxifylline in granulomatous diseases. Thalidomide, which is presently used to treat some forms of leprosy, has also been shown to specifically inhibit transcription of the TNF gene in monocytes[52].

- **Anti interleukin-2 receptor and interleukin-1ß treatment**

As shown in fig.1 interleukin-1 (IL-1) and interleukin-2 (IL-2) play a role in HLA class II restricted antigen presentation and (auto-)immune response. This is confirmed in IBD by studies showing enhanced IL-2 and IL-1ß production[53] in mononuclear cells isolated from the mucosa and biopsy specimens[17]. In autoimmune diseases and in Crohn's disease serum soluble IL-2 receptor concentration is raised, indicating T-cell19. Intestinal mucosal mononuclear cells of Crohn's disease patients produce only one-third of the amount of interleukin-2 generated by control cells after stimulation, but were able to exhibit comparable cytotoxicity[54]. This is probably due to either an increased number of interleukin-2 responsive cells or an exaggerated reactivity to interleukin-2. Lack of IL-2 production seems to play a role in the disability of a granulomatous response to Schistosoma mansoni in mice[55]. Recombinant IL-2 therapy reversed this diminished response. Its not clear what the exact function of the granuloma formation in Crohn's disease is; Is it an exaggerated immune response to antigens or a decreased response to bacteria? Counteracting IL-2 production or neutralizing its effects by monoclonal antibodies directed against its receptor, may be an option for immunotherapy of Crohn's disease especially when we consider the antigen c.q. abnormal immune response. Monoclonal antibodies against IL-2 receptor are used in the prophylactic treatment of human kidney allograft recipients, with good result and only few side effects[56]. No studies are as yet available on monoclonal antibody treatment against the IL-1 receptor.

REFERENCES

1 Katz KD, Hollander D, Vadheim CM, et al. Intestinal permeability in patients with Crohn's disease and their healthy relatives. Gastroenterology 1989;97:927-31.

2 Howden CW, Robertson C, Ducan A, Morris AJ, Russel RI. Comparison of different measurements of intestinal permeability in inflammatory bowel disease. Am J Gastroenterol 1991;86:1445-9.

3 Madara JL, Moore R, Carlson S. Alteration of intestinal tight junction structure and permeability by cytoskeletal contraction. Am Phy Soc 1987;C854-61.

4 Ouyang Q, El-Youssef M, Yen-Lieberman B, Sapatnekar W, Youngman KR, Kusugami K, et al. Expression of HLA-DR antigens in inflammatory bowel disease mucosa: Role of intestinal lamina propria mononuclear cell-derived interferon τ. Dig Dis Sci 1988;33:1528-36.

5 Cuvelier C, Mielants H, Vos de M, Veys E, Roels H. Major histocompatibility complex class II antigen (HLA-DR) expression by ileal epithelial cells in patients with seronegative spondylarthropathy. Gut 1990;31:545-9.

6 Mayer L, Eisenhardt D, Salomon P, Bauer W, Plous R, Piccinini L. Expression of class II molecules on intestinal epithelial cells in humans. Differences between normal and inflammatory bowel diseases. Gastroenterology 1991;100:3-12.

7 James SP, Fiocchi C, Greaff AS, Strober W. Phenotypic analysis of lamina propria lymphocytes. Predominance of helper-inducer and cytolytic T-cell phenotypes and deficiency of suppressor-inducer phenotypes in Crohn's disease and controle patients. Gastroenterology 1986;91:1483-9.

8 Rappaport H, Burgoyne FH, Smetana HF. The pathology of regional enteritis. Milit Surg 1951;109:463-502

9 Zifronini A, Treves AJ, Sachar DB, Rachmilewitz D. Prostanoid synthesis by cultured intestinal epithelial and mononuclear cells in inflammatory bowel disease. Gut 1983;24:659-65.

10 Ferguson A. Why study T cell subsets in Crohn's disease? Gut 1983;24:687-91.
11 Selby WS, Janossy G, Bofill M, Jewell DP. Intestinal lymphocyte subpopulations in inflammatory bowel disease: an analysis by immunohistological and cell isolation techniques. Gut 1984;25:32-40.
12 Konttinen YT, Bergroth V, Nordstrom D, Segerberg-Konttinen M, Seppala K, Salaspuro M. Lymphocyte activation in vivo in the intestinal mucosa of patients with Crohn's disease. J Clin Lab Immunol 1987;22:59-63.
13 Fais S, Pallone F, Squarcia O, et al. HLA-DR antigens on colonic epithelial cells in inflammatory bowel disease: 1. Relation to the state of activation of lamina propria lymphocytes and to the epithelial expression of other surface markers. Clin Exp Immunol 1987;68:605-12.
14 Pallone F, Fais S, Squarcia O, Biancone L, Pozzilli P, Boivirant M. Activation of peripheral blood and intestinal lamina propria lymphocytes in Crohn's disease. In vivo state of activation and in vitro response to stimulation as defined by expression of early activation antigens. Gut 1987;28:745-53.
15 Choy MY, Walker-Smith JA, Williams CB, MacDonald TT. Differential expression of CD25 (interleukin-2 receptor) on lamina propria T cells and macrophages in the intestinal lesions in Crohn's disease and ulcerative colitis. Gut 1990;31:1365-70.
16 Monk TJ, Spencer J, Cerf-Bensussan N, MacDonald TT. Activation of mucosal T-cells in situ with anti-CD3 antibody: phenotype of activated T-cells and their distribution within the mucosal micro-environment. Clin Exp Immunol 1988;74:216-22.
17 Brynskov J, Tvede N, Andersen CB, Vilien M. Increased concentrations of interleukin 1ß,, interleukin-2, and soluble interleukin-2 receptors in endoscopic mucosal biopsy specimens with active inflammatory bowel disease. Gut 1992;33:55-58.
18 Meuler CH, Knoflach P, Zielinski CC. T-cell activation in Crohn's disease. Gastroenterology 1990;98:639-46.
19 Crabtree JE, Juby LD, Heatley RV, Lobo AJ, Bullimore DW, Axon ATR. Soluble interleukin-2 receptor in Crohn's disease: relation of serum concentrations to disease activity. Gut 1990;31:1033-6.
20 Mahida YR, Callager A, Kurlak L, Hawkey CY. Plasma and tissue interleukin-2 receptor level in IBD. Clin Exp Immunol 1990;82:75-80.
21 Senju M, Hulstaert F, Lowder J, Jewell DP. Flow cytometric analysis of peripheral blood lymphocytes in ulcerative colitis and Crohn's disease. Gut 1991;32:779-83.
22 Cher DJ, Mosman TR. Two types of murine T cell clone. II. Delayed type hypersensitivity is mediated by Th1 clones. J Immunol 1987;138:3688-94.
23 Ashwell DJ, Fox BS, Schwartz RH. T cell recognition of antigen and Ia molecules involves a trimolecular complex. in Processing and presentation of antigens 1988;Academic Press, Inc London
24 Stewart-Tull DES. Immunologically important constituents of mycobacteria: adjuvants. in Biology of Mycobacteria Vol 2.1983 Academic Press London. IBSN 0-12-582302-9.

25 Blaauwgeers JL, Das PK, Slob AW, Houthoff HJ. Human gut wall reactivity to monoclonal antibodies against M. avium glycolipid in relation to Crohn's disease (preliminary results). Acta Leprol (Geneve) 1989;7 Suppl 1:138-40.
26 Thayer WR Jr, Coutu JA, Chiodini RJ, Van Kruiningen HJ, Merkal RS. Possible role of mycobacteria in inflammatory bowel disease. II. Mycobacterial antibodies in Crohn's disease. Dig Dis Sci 1984;29:1080-5.
27 Haanen JBAG, Waal de Malefijt R, Res PCM, Kraakman EM, Ottenhof THM, Vries RRP, et al. Selection of a human T helper type 1-like T cell subset by mycobacteria. J Exp Med 1991;174:583-92.
28 Ebert EC, Bhatt BD, Lui S, Das KM. Induction of suppressor cells by Mycobacterium paratuberculosis antigen in inflammatory bowel disease. Cli Exp Immunol 1991;83:320-5.
29 Atalla L, Linker-Israeli M, Steinman L, Rao NA. Inhibition of autoimmune uveitis by Anti-CD4 antibody. Invest Ophthalmol Vis Sci 1990;31:1264-70.
30 Hafler DA, Fallis RJ, Dawson DM, Schlossman SF, Reinherz EL, Weiner HL. Immunologic responses of progressive multiple sclerosos patients treated with an anti-T-cell monoclonal antibody, anti-T12. Neurol 1986;36:777-84.
31 Ortho Multicenter Transplantation Group. N Eng J Med 1985;313:337-42.
32 Ziegler EJ,. N Eng J Med 1991;324:429-.
33 Catane R, Longo DL. Isr J Med Sci 1988;24:471-.
34 O'Brien JJ, Bayless TM, Bayless JA. Use of Azathioprine or 6-Mercaptopurine in treatment of Crohn's disease. Gastroenterology 1991;101:39-46.
35 Hess AD, Colombani PM. Cyclosporin: mechanism of action: *in vitro* studies. Prog Allergy 1986;38:198-221.
36 Brynskov J, Freund L, Rasmussen SN, Lauritsen K, Schaffalitzky de Muckadell O, Williams N, et al. A placebo-controlled, double-blind, randomized trial of cyclosporine therapy in active chronic Crohn's disease. N Engl J Med 1989;321:845-50
37 Alters SE, Sakai K, Steinman L, Oi VT. Mechanisms of anti-CD-mediated depletion and immunotherapy. A study using a set of chimeric anti-CD4 antibodies. J Immunol 1990;144:4587-92.
38 James SP. Remission of Crohn's disease after human immunodeficiency virus infection. Gastroenterology 1988;95:1667-9.
39 Herzog C, Walker C, Müller W, Rieber P, Reiter C,Rietmüller G, et al. Anti-CD4 antibody treatment of patients with Rheumatoid arthritis: I. Effect on clinical course and circulating T Cells. J Autoimmunity 1998;2:627-42
40 Walker C, Herzog C, Rieber P, Rietmüller G, Müller W, Pichler WJ. Anti-CD4 antibody treatment of patients with reumatoid arthritis: II. Effect of *in vivo* treatment on *in vitro* proliverative response of CD4 cells. J Autoimmun 1989;2:643-9.
41 Asano M, Minagawa T, Ohamichi M, Hiraga Y. Detection of endogenous cytokines in sera or lymph nodes obtained from patients with

sarcoidosis. Clin Exp Immunol 1991:84:92-6.
42 Ruco LP; Stoppacciaro A; Pomponi D; Boraschi D; Santoni A; Tagliabue A; Uccini S; Baroni CD. Immunoreactivity for IL-1 beta and TNF alpha in human lymphoid and nonlymphoid tissues. Am J Pathol 1989;135:889-97.
43 Dunn CJ, Hardee MM, Staite ND. Acute and chronic inflammatory responses to local administration of recombinant IL-1 alpha, IL-beta, TNF alpha, IL-2 and Ifn gamma in mice. Agents Actions 1989;27:290-3.
44 Kindler V, Sappino AP, Grau G, Piguet PF, Vassalli P. The inducing role of tumor necrosis factor in the development of bactericidal granulomas during BCG infection. Cell 1989;56:731-40.
45 MacDonald TT, Hutchings P, Choy M-Y, Murch S, Cooke A. Tumor necrosis factor-alpha and interferon-gamma production measured at the single cell level in normal and inflamed human intestine. Cli Exp Immunol 1990;81:301-5.
46 Braegger CP, Nicholls S, Murch SH, Stephens S, MacDonald TT. Tumour necrosis factor alpha in stool as a marker of intestinal inflammation. Lancet 1992;339:89-91.
47 Exley AR, Cohen J, Buurman W, et al. Monoclonal antibody to TNF in severe septic shock. Lancet 1990;335:1275-7.
48 Schönharting MM, Schade UF. The effect of pentoxyfilline in septic shock - new pharmacological aspects of an established drug. J Med 1989;20:97-105.
49 Schade UF. Pentoxyfylline increases survival in murine endotoxine shock and decreases formation of tumor necrosis factor.Circ Shock 1990;31:171-81.
50 Strieter RM, Remick DG, Ward PA et al. Cellular and molecular regulation of tumor necrosis factor-alpha production by pentoxyfilline. Biochem Biophys Res Comm 1988;155:1230-6.
51 Sullivan GW, Carper HT, Novick WJ, Mandell GL. Inhibition of inflammatory action of interleukin-1 and tumor necrosis factor (alpha) on neutrophil function by Pentoxifylline. Infect Immun 1988;56:1722-9.
52 Sampaio EP, Sarno EN, Galilly R, Kaplan G. Thalidomide selectively inhibits tumor necrosis factor alpha production by stimulated human monocytes. J Exp Med 1991;173:699-703.
53 Mahida YR, Wu K, Jewel DP. Enhanced production of interleukin 1-ß by mononuclear cells isolated from mucosa with active ulcerative colitis or Crohn's disease. Gut 1989;30:835-8.
54 Kusugami K, Youngman KR, West GA, Fiocchi C. Intestinal immune reactivity to interleukin 2 differs among Crohn's disease, ulcerative colitis. and controls. Gastroenterology 1989;97:1-9.
55 Mathew RC, Ragheb S, Boros DL. Recombinant IL-2 therapy reverses diminished granulomatous responsiveness in anti-L3T4-treated, *Schistosoma mansoni*-infected mice. J Immunol 1990;144:4356-61.
56 Peyronnet P, Le Mauff B, Hourmant M, Cantarovich D, Dudigeon P, Olive D, et al. Prophylactic treatment of human kidney allograft recipients with a monoclonal antibody (33B3.1) directed against interleukin 2 receptor. Transplantation Procedings 1988;20:300-2.

IS IMMUNOTHERAPY WITH MYCOBACTERIUM VACCAE APPROPRIATE TO CROHN'S DISEASE?

John L. Stanford

Department of Medical Microbiology School of Pathology University College and Middlesex School of Medicine 67-73, Riding House Street London W1P 7LD, UK.

INTRODUCTION

It is highly likely that the inflammatory bowel diseases are all infections, but the question remains as to the identity of the causative organism or organisms. Accepting that they are infections is more important than knowing the identity of the organisms themselves, or knowing the precise genetic makeup of persons whose response to such infections will be to develop these diseases. Their aetiology is likely to be bacterial rather than viral, and for a number of reasons these bacteria are unlikely to be present in the tissues in their conventional form. The very slow progression of these diseases in most cases, their very slow response to antibacterial agents, and the difficulty experienced in demonstrating them in the tissues all suggest that the pathology of the disease is an excessive response to a small number of very slowly growing organisms for which the term "slow bacteria" seems appropriate (1).

There are a number of diseases for which such a slow bacterial aetiology seems probable. These include sarcoidosis, rheumatoid arthritis and psoriasis as well as inflammatory bowel disease, for all of which an increase in agalactosyl immunoglobulin levels seems to be a marker (2). This aberrant form of IgG is also raised in tuberculosis and at certain times in leprosy. It appears to be both a marker for these infections and for the type of T-lymphocyte mediated tissue damage accompanied by an acute phase response that typifies the immunpathological response constituting the lesions (3).

An individual propensity for developing disease in response to infectious challenge with these organisms is likely to depend on his or her genetic makeup and environmental experience. Thus the epidemiological approach to confirm that Crohn's disease or ulcerative colitis are infections has not been easy. However, it must be remembered that neither tuberculosis nor leprosy were generally recognized as infections until the causative organisms were demonstrated.

ARE CROHN'S DISEASE AND ULCERATIVE COLITIS DIFFERENT EXPRESSIONS OF THE SAME DISEASE?

The demonstration that leprosy was a disease with a wide spectrum of immunopathology, with the multibacillary lepromatous form at one end and the paucibacillary tuberculoid form at the other, has had a profound effect on conceptual frameworks for helping to understand disease (4). It has both helped in explaining how infection with a single bacterial species can give rise to different syndromes of disease due to different immunological responses, and hindered in obscuring spectra based on toher aspects. Although much less wellknown, tropical ulcerative mycobacteriosis, Buruli ulcer, or Mycobacterium ulcerans infection also have a disease spectrum, but one through which each sufferer passes, from the multibacillary immunosuppressive tissue necrotic phase to the paucibacillary granulomatous fibrotic healing phase (5). In the inflammatory bowel diseases the spectrum may be due to locally different expressions of immune response to the same infectious agent taking place in different tissues. Thus the lesions of intestinal tuberculosis in man are often different when they occur in the terminal ileum from when they occur in the colon. The majority of ileal tuberculosis is granulomatous, whereas colonic tuberculosis is ofter ulcerative with little or no granuloma formation (6).

WHAT ARE THE ORGANISMS CAUSING CROHN'S DISEASE AND ULCERATIVE COLITIS?

This is not yet the time to argue for or against a particular view, or particular results, but to record observations and await developments. I have been fortunate in my laboratory to work with Professor Lennard Jones, Dr Burnham. Dr White, Dr Visuvanathan and Mr McIntyre over a period extending from 1978 until now. During this time we have carried out 2 blinded surveys of bacteriological isolation of unusual bacteria from lymh nodes draining bowel affected with Crohn's disease, ulcerative colitis or unrelated diseases. The results obtained in the two surveys have been essentially the same (7,8,9 and see the table).

TABLE

Table showing isolations of pleomorphic acid fast bacteria form lymph node tissue draining the bowel.

	1978 series	1988 series
Crohn's disease	42/76 (55%) P < 0.00001	17/25 (68%) P < 0.002
Other conditions (controls)	3/41 (7%) P < 0.00001	3/17 (18%) P = 0.002
Ulcerative colitis	14/27 (52%)	11/15 (73%)

All positive cultures were obtained on Robertson's cooked meat medium, after 3 months to 18 months at 32°C.

Although we still do not have a definitive identity for the organsisms isolated, a solid body of information about them is building up. The organisms are pleomorphic, variably acid-fast, possess traces of tuberculostearic acid and mycolic acid, but lack lipoarabinomannan in their cell walls. Related to mycobacteria, but perhaps better thought of as near-mycobacteria at this stage, their genetic identity is not yet fully confirmed. Producing positive dot blots with some mycobacterial gene probes, and the majority of them appearing homologous, their final identity may come from the sequencing that is currently in progress. A number of these isolates have been passaged through nude mize by Drs McDermott and Banerjee, and slowly growing conventional mycobacteria have been isolated from their tissues, bringing to mind the studies of Mitchell and Rees (10).

IMMUNOTHERAPY WITH MYCOBACTERIUM VACCAE AND ITS POTENTIAL ISE IN INFLAMMATORY BOWEL DISEASE

Although under ideal conditions the currently availlable chemotherapy with 3 or 4 effective drugs is capable of successfully curing both leprosy and tuberculosis with few failures, worldwide perspectives show results less impressive. In leprosy, reactions continue do destroy nerves and faces long after effective antibacterial treatment has begun, or even been completed. In tuberculosis, costs of drugs, their administration and overcoming patient non-compliance, compounded by increasing levels of bacterial drug resistance, aspecially to rifampicin and isoniazid, and now, devastatingly, by HIV infection, have led to a breakdown in control. The need for shorter and more effective treatments which might overcome drug resistance has led to a return to ideas of treatments based on stimulation of the immune system to destroy bacteria. Such an approach is especially suitable for mycobacterial diseases, and to those caused by the putative slow bacteria for the following reasons.

1 Slowly metabolizing and multiplying bacteria require long periods of chemotherapy, since the antibacterial mechanisms of action of the drugs work by interference in the processes.
2 Bacterial persistance, or the ability to remain live but resting in the tissues, and therefore in a state protected from antibacterial action of drugs, is typical of mycobacteria, and probably of other slow bacteria.
3 The immunological pathway of the Koch phenomenon in which antigens presented by cells to T lymphocytes leads to their release of cytokines resulting in tissue death, is not the optimal mechanism for bacterial killing (11).

The principle of immunotherapy is to induce recognition of even resting bacteria by their surface antigens, and to promote their killing by immune mechanisms. This requires both the enhancement of surface antigen recognition, and the replacement of T cell mediated tissue destruction by the true mechanism of protective immunity in which invading bacteria are killed. This latter should be accompanied by a return to normal levels of circulating agalactosyl immunoglobulin.

Studies over many years have shown that suspensions of a killed, selected, strain of the harmless environmental saprophyte Mycobacterium vaccae, has both the required properties (12). A single intradermal injection of this suspension, used as an adjunct to antibacterial chemotherapy is proving very effective in established mycobacterial disease. Thus it doubles the rate of removal of leprosy bacilli in newly diagnosed mutlibacillary leprosy, and it inncreased the rate of disappearance of tubercle bacilli from the sputum of patients with pulmonary tuberculosis in an on-going study in Nigeria (13). In a controlled and blinded trial in The Gambia, immunotherapy with M. vaccae significantly reduced mortality over an 18 month follow-up period in patients who were considered to have complied with chemotherapy (14). In this study the level of agalactosyl IgG fell significantly faster in the recipients of the immunotherapy than in the recipients of placebo. Open studies of its use in the retreatment of treament failures due to drug resistance in tuberculosis have shown immunotherapy with M. vaccae to lead to substained disappearance of bacilli from the sputum, resolution of signs and relief of symptoms in patients in India, Iran, Romania, Vietnam and the United Kingdom.

Currently being tried in a number of diseases of uncertain aaetiology, a number of dramatic, but still anecdotal, successes have been recorded. In psoriasis immunotherapy with M. vaccae has recently been found to be very effective in a group of Indian patients (15), and similar results have been achieved in on-going studies in Argentina, Iran and the United Kingdom. Although no studies have started yet in Crohn's disease, with its excessive granuloma formation and increased level of agalactosyl IgG, this is exactly the type of disease that might be expected to respond to such treatment. At the moment more than 10.000 people have received injections of killed M. vaccae as part of programmes of immunoprophylaxis or immunotherapy, with no more serious side effects than those accompanying BCG vaccination of a British school child.

It is difficult to see how much attempted immunotherapy could be harmful, and the potential benefit for the patient is enormous. Data obtained from patients with rheumatoid arthritis suggest that immunosuppressive drugs may be prejudicial to immunotherapeutic succes, and therefore it might be better employ M. vaccae during a period of remission, rather than at a time when symptomatic suppression is required. An initial open study could be simple with a randomized half of a group of patients with quiescent Crohn's disease being give the injection. Follow-up might record relapses, assessments of symptomatic wellbeing, and the level of circulating agalactosyl immunoglobulin.

REFERENCES

1 Rook GAW, Stanford JL. autoimmunity or slow bacterial infections? Immunology Today 1992 (in press).

2 Dude R, Rook GAW, Steele J, Brealey R, Dwek R, Rademacher T, Lennard-Jones J. Agalactosyl IgG in inflammatory bowel disease: correlation with C-reactive protein. Gut 1990;31:431-434.

3 Rook GAW, Al-Attiyah R. Cytokines and the Koch Phenomenon. Tubercle 1991;72:13-20.

4 Ridley DS, Jopling WH. Classification of leprosy according to immunity. A five group system. International Journal of Leprosy 1966;34:255-273.

5 Stanford JL, Hutt MSR, Phillips I, Revill WDL. Antibiotic treatment in Mycobacterium ulcerans infection. Ain Shams Medical Journal 1974;25:suppl.5;258-261.

6 Vij JC. Personal communication.

7 Butnham WR, Lennard-Jones JE, Stanford JL, Bird RJ. Mycobacteria as a possible cause of inflammatory bowel disease.. Lancet 1978;2:693-696.

8 Stanford JL, Dourmashkin R, McIntyre G. An investigation into the role of mycobacteria in Crohn's disease.
In "Inflammatory bowel disease - frontiers in aetiology". 1978. Proceedings of the 8th BSG/SK & F International Workshop 24-28.
9 Visuvanathan S. The characterization of pleomorphic acid fast organisms isolated from patients with imflammatory bowel disease.
MD thesis, University of London. 1990.
10 Mitchell DN, Ress RJW. Agent transmissible from Crohn's disease tissue.
Lancet 1970;2:1680171.
11 Stanford JL. Koch's phenomenon, can it be corrected?
Tubercle 1991;72: in press.
12 Stanford jl, Rook GAW, Bahr GM, Dowlati Y, Ganapati R, Ghazi Saidi K, Lucas S, Ramu G, Torres P, Ho Monh Ly, Anstey N. Mycobacterium vaccae in immunoporphylaxis and immunotherapy of leprosy and tuberculosis.
Vaccine 1990;8:525-530.
13 Onyebujoh P, Rook GAW. Mycobacterium vaccae immunotherapy.
Lancet 1991;338:letter p.1534.
14 Corrah PT, Byass P, Stanford JL, Thomas V, Bouchier V, Whittle HC. The effects of prios vaccination with BCG and of immunotherapy on the outcome of treatment for pulmonary tuberculosis (in preparation). 1992.
15 Ramu G, Prema GD, Balakrishnan S, Shanker Narayan NP, Stanford JL. A preliminary report on the immunotherapy of psoriasis.
Indian Medical Gazette 1990;124:381-382.

MYCOBACTERIAL ETIOLOGY OF CROHN'S DISEASE: HOW TO PROVE CAUSATION

Fouad A.K. El-Zaatari, Ph.D
David Y. Graham, M.D.

Inflammatory Bowel Disease Laboratory Veterans Affairs Medical Center and Departments of Medicine and Molecular Virology Baylor College of Medicine Houston, Texas, U.S.A.

INTRODUCTION

It has long been suspected that the inflammatory bowel diseases, ulcerative colitis and Crohn's disease, have infectious etiologies. Over the last 60 years, there have been a number of candidate etiologic agents for each disease (1). Recent evidence has focused on a mycobacterial etiology. In 1932, Crohn, Oppenheimer, and Ginzburg separated Crohn's disease from intestinal tuberculosis caused by Mycobacterium tuberculosis (2) but interest in a possible etiologic role of other mycobacteria in Crohn's disease continued. Provocative results were produced from several laboratories but no real progress was made until the isolation of what were initially described as uncharacterized mycobacteria from 2 tissues from patients with Crohn's disease (3). The incubation periods were quite long and each isolate went through a cell-wall defective phase before reverting to traditionally cultivatable mycobacteria. These organisms were initially isolated as cell-wall defective organisms and were very fastidious (4-6). Our group was the first to identify the isolates as M. paratuberculosis and this has been confirmed (7,8). Since then a series of papers describing the isolation of M. paratuberculosis from Crohn's disease patients have been published (9-11). M. paratuberculosis is the cause of a chronic intestinal disease in animals (similar to Crohn's in humans) called ruminant paratuberculosis or Johne's disease and also has been associated with gastrointestinal disease in primates (12,13). These reports rekindled interest in a mycobacterial etiology for Crohn's disease because they provided plausible explanations (extreme fastidiousness due to existence as cell-wall defective organisms and to mycobactin dependence) for difficulties previously encountered in culturing mycobacteria from involved tissues.

It has become apparent that mycobacteria are not recovered exclusively from Crohn's disease tissues. We isolated mycobacteria from intestinal specimens obtained by surgical resection or endoscopic biopsy from patients with Crohn's disease, those with ulcerative colitis, and non-inflammatory bowel disease controls (5,6,14). Conventional mycobacteria and spheroplasts (cell wall-defective forms) were isolated from approximately one-third of the patients in each group studied. Many isolates, particularly those from resected tissue specimens, appear to be cell wall-defective when first isolated.

The similarity of Crohn's disease to Johne's disease caused by M. paratuberculosis and the recovery of M. paratuberculosis from Crohn's disease tissues is very provocative. While it is clear that M. paratuberculosis can be cultured from some patients with Crohn's disease, the picture is clouded by the fact that mycobacteria can also be cultured from intestinal tissues from patients with ulcerative colitis and even from patients with no evidence of inflammatory bowel disease. This suggests that mycobacteria are commonly present as part of the normal microflora of the gut. Furthermore, nucleic acid hybridization experiments have shown that mycobacterial DNA is often present within the intestinal muscle layers of patients with Crohn's disease (indicating that the mycobacteria were not luminal contaminants). However, these studies also showed that mycobacterial DNA was present in patients with ulcerative colitis and in normal controls (7).

Until recently, we found it impossible to identify the spheroplasts as mycobacteria and to discern whether they were the same species. We have now been able to accomplish this using the polymerase chain reaction (PCR) based on the presence of an insertion sequence (IS900) in M. paratuberculosis (15). This insertion element (1.4Kb) is thought to be present in all M. paratuberculosis (16,17) and absent from M. avium genomic DNA. Sequences different but related to IS900 (IS902) have been found in some mycobactin-dependent M. avium isolated from the Wood pigeon which also causes chronic enteritis in calves (16-18). Subsequently, the nucleotide sequences of the IS900, and the related IS902 element from M. avium have been determined (16,17). In collaboration of Professor Hermon-Taylor's group (St. George's Hospital, University of London, London, U.K.), specific DNA probes were used to identify our isolates and 75% (6 of 8) of our positive isolates (by culture and PCR) that were primarily isolated as spheroplasts from patients with Crohn's disease are M. paratuberculosis; isolates from patients with ulcerative colitis and non-inflammatory bowel disease controls that were isolated primarily as spheroplasts have not been M. paratuberculosis; one slow grower that was not isolated as spheroplast from a non-inflammatory bowel disease biopsy was M. paratuberculosis (19). The frequency of M. paratuberculosis (our data plus that from other laboratories) from Crohn's disease was significantly greater than from ulcerative colitis or non-inflammatory bowel disease controls [5 of 40 (12.5%) controls versus 26 of 40 (65%) Crohn's disease tissue specimens, $p < 0.001$; (20 and Hermon-Taylor, personal communication)]. Improved cultural techniques and the use of specific primers in PCR-based assays have strengthened the association of M. paratuberculosis and Crohn's disease.

Although PCR will continue to be invaluable to strengthen the association of M. paratuberculosis to Crohn's disease, PCR alone will not provide data critical to understanding how it may be involved. As shown above, M. paratuberculosis is present in tissues of patients with Crohn's disease. We believe this is as a cell-wall deficient form with low multiplication that persists within the infected intestinal tissues and is responsible for triggering an abnormal and/or continuing immune or autoimmune response which leads to the disease. This by no means indicates that M. paratuberculosis per se are the sole and complete causative events of disease, but rather other environmental and/or genetic factor(s) may facilitate it's establishment, persistence, and production of disease.

The fact that these organisms are in the tissues as spheroplasts coupled with the availability of mycobacteria- specific probes will allow their detection and specific localization within the gut wall by the in situ hybridization technique. In situ hybridization not only will allow detection but will also show whether the M. paratuberculosis are associated with disease and granulomas within disease tissues. Their presence as spheroplasts will enhance the ease of detection as it is very difficult to lyse mycobacteria without destroying structures. Detection of M. paratuberculosis variants or materials within the gut wall would be an enormous step forward in search of an etiological agent in Crohn's disease. Demonstration that mycobacteria, even better a specific Mycobacterium, are invariably associated with the granulomas of Crohn's disease would be compelling evidence for a critical role of mycobacteria in the pathogenesis of the disease.

Over a decade of research has been directed at the laboratory culture of Mycobacteria and spheroplasts of uncertain nature from patients with Crohn's disease. With the advent of molecular cloning, monoclonal antibodies, T-cell cloning, and the PCR methods, scientists have been able to identify some of the immunodominant proteins from some of the most puzzling and complex disease agents, M. leprae and M. tuberculosis. Cloning the genomes of these organisms in expression vectors and propagating pathogen-specific T cell clones isolated from patients has had a major impact in mycobacteria research. Screening of M. tuberculosis, M. bovis/BCG, and M. leprae in gt11 and in plasmid libraries with rabbit hyperimmune sera and Murine monoclonal antibodies produced several antibody binding clones (21-24). A series of proteins known as 70K, 65K, 36K, 30K, 31K, 28K 18K and 12K antigens from M. leprae have been identified and subsequently some of their nucleotide sequences and their B- and T cell epitopes have been published (25,26). The diagnostic potential and their possible role of these proteins in the immune response are now being determined (27,28). Some of these proteins were originally identified with leprosy and tuberculosis patient sera (26,29), however, disease-specific associations required analysis of responses to T cell and B cell epitopes produced in expression libraries. Future studies based on using similar molecular biology strategies successfully applied to M. tuberculosis, M. leprae and M. bovis/BCG should help answer whether there is a disease-specific association of Mycobacterium paratuberculosis and Crohn's disease. Well-defined recombinant antigens representing the M. isolates will be useful tools for the localization of both B and T cell epitopes. Understanding the chemical nature of these determinants and amino acid motifs on the isolated organisms should facilitate the development of specific diagnostic tests and investigation of their role in protective immunity and pathogenesis of disease.

Definitive evidence of a mycobacterial agent, specifically M. paratuberculosis, as critically involved in the pathogenesis of Crohn's disease is lacking but the absence of a satisfactory alternative etiology and the availability of methods that can definitively answer the question justifies consideration of this possible association. Most investigators now believe that Crohn's disease is the product of a sustained immunological response to a persisting antigen. Mycobacteria live within macrophages, and it would not be unreasonable that a number of different mycobacterial species might cause the same process in different individuals who are appropriately immunologically primed. The possibility that M. paratuberculosis is not the sole cause of Crohn's disease should not curtail studies of microbial involvement in the pathogenesis of Crohn's disease; rather, it suggests that the problem will be more difficult to unravel than some would hope. We now have the techniques to prove whether M. paratuberculosis is etiologically related to Crohn's disease; we believe the answer will be "yes".

REFERENCES

1 Graham DY, Markesich DC, Yoshimura HH, Estes MK. Microbial aetiology of Crohn's disease: mycobacteria - cause or commensal? In: Inflammatory Bowel Disease. AA Anagnostides, HJF Hodgson, JB Kirsner (Eds). Chapman & Hall Medical, New York, 1991; pp 179-200.

2 Crohn BB, Ginzburg L, Oppenheimer GD. Regional ileitis. A pathologic and clinical entity. JAMA 1932;99:1323-1329.

3 Chiodini RJ, Van Kruiningen HJ, Thayer WR, et al. Possible role of mycobacteria in inflammatory bowel disease. I. An unclassified Mycobacterium species isolated from patients with Crohn's disease. Dig Dis Sci 1984;29:1073-9.

4 Chiodini RJ, Van Kruiningen HJ, Thayer WR, et al. Spheroplastic phase of mycobacteria isolated from patients with Crohn's disease. J Clin Microbiol 1986;27:357-63.

5 Graham DY, Markesich DC, Yoshimura HH. Mycobacteria and inflammatory bowel disease: results of culture. Gastroenterology 1987;92:436-42.
6 Markesich DC, Graham DY, Yoshimura HH. Progress in culture/subculture of spheroplasts and fastidious acid-fast bacilli isolated from intestinal tissues. J Clin Microbiol 1988:26;1600-3.
7 Yoshimura HH, Graham DY, Estes MK, et al. Investigation of association of mycobacteria with inflammatory bowel disease by nucleic acid hybridization. J Clin Microbiol 1987;25:45-51.
8 McFadden JJ, Butcher PD, Chiodini RJ, Hermon-Taylor J. Crohn's disease-isolated mycobacteria are identical to Mycobacterium paratuberculosis, as determined by DNA probes that distinguish between mycobacterial species. J Clin Microbiol 1987;25:796-801.
9 Haagsma J, Mulder CJJ, Eger A, Bruins J, Ketel RJ, Tytgat GNJ. Mycobacterium species isolated from patients with Crohn's Disease. IN: Inflammatory Bowel Disease: current status and future approach. MacDermott RP (Ed.), Elsevier Science Publishers B.V., Amsterdam, 1988, pp. 535-7.
10 McFadden JJ, Thompson J, Green E, Hampson SJ, Stanford J, Haagsma J, Chiodini R, Hermon-Taylor J. Indentification and characterization of further bacteria isolated from Crohn's disease and control tissues. Gastroenterology 1988;94:A294.
11 Gitnick G, Collins J, Beaman B, Brooks D, Arthur M, Imaeda T, Palieschesky M. Preliminary report on isolation of mycobacteria from patients with Crohn's disease. Dig Dis Sci 1989;34:925-32.
12 Chiodini RJ, Van Kruiningen HJ, and Merkal RS. Ruminant paratuberculosis (Johne's disease): the current status and future prospects. Cornell Vet 1984;74:218-62.
13 McClure HM, Chiodini RJ, Anderson DC, et al. M. paratuberculosis (Johne's disease) in a colony of stump-tail macaques (Macaca arctoides). J Infect Dis 1987;155:1011-1019.
14 Markesich DC, Graham DY, Yoshimura HH. Progress in culture and subculture of spheroplasts and fastidious acid bacilli isolated from intestinal tissues. J Clin Microbiol 1988; 26:1600-3.
15 Green EP, Tizard MLV, Moss MT, et al. Sequence and characteristics of 1S900, an insertion element identified in a human Crohn's disease isolate of Mycobacterium paratuberculosis. Nucleic Acid Res 1989;17:9063-73.
16 Hermon-Taylor J, Moss M, Tizard M, Sanderson J. Molecular biology of Crohn's disease mycobacteria. Bailliere's Clin Gastroenterol 1990;4:23-42.
17 Vary PH, Anderson PR, Green E, Hermon-Taylor J, McFadden JJ. Use of highly specific DNA probes and the PCR to detect Mycobacterium paratuberculosis in Johne's disease. J Clin Microbiol 1990;28:933-937.
18 Moss MT, Green EP, Tizard ML, Malik ZP, Hermon-Taylor J. Specific detection of M. paratuberculosis by DNA hybridization with a fragment of the insertion element IS900. Gut 1991;32:395-398.
19 Moss M T, Sanderson J D, Tizard MLV, et al. M. paratuberculosis in long term cultures of Crohn's disease tissues revealed by PCR amplification of IS900. Gastroenterology 1991;100:A232.

20 Sanderson JD, Moss MT, Tizard MLV, Green EP and Hermon-Taylor J. PCR detection of M. paratuberculosis in Crohn's disease tissues DNA extracts. Gastroenterology 1991;100:A44.

21 Young RA, Mehra V, Sweetser D, et al. Genes for the major protein antigens of the leprosy parasite Mycobacterium leprae. Nature 1985;316:450-2.

22 Young RA, Bloom BR, Crosskimsky CM, et al. Dissection of Mycobacterium tuberculosis antigens using recombinant DNA. Proc Natl Acad Sci USA 1985;82:2583-7.

23 Thole JR, Danwese HG, Das PK, et al. Cloning of Mycobacterium bovis BCG DNA and expression of antigens in E. Coli. Infect Immun 1985;50:800-6.

24 Hopwood DA, Kieser T, Colston MJ, et al. Molecular biology of Mycobacteria. Brit Med Bul 1988;44:528-46.

25 Young DB. Structure of mycobacterial antigens. Brit Med Bul 1988;44:562-83.

26 Watson JD. Leprosy: understanding protective immunity. Immunol Today 1989;10:218-21.

27 Williams DL, Gillis TP, Booth RJ, et al. The use of a specific probe and PCR for the detection of M. leprae. J Infect Dis 1990;162:193-200.

28 Mustafa AS, Gill HK, Nerland A, et al. Human T-cell clones recognize a major M. leprae protein antigen expressed in E. coli. Nature 1986;319:63-68.

29 Hartskeerl RA, Ren RMV, Stabel LFEM, et al. Selection and characterization of recombinant clones that produce M. leprae antigens recognized by antibodies in sera from household contacts of leprosy patients. Infect Immun 1990;58:2821-2827.

Developments in Gastroenterology

1. A. S. Peña, I.T. Weterman, C.C. Booth and W. Strober (eds.): *Recent Advances in Crohn's Disease*. Proceedings of the 2nd International Workshop on Crohn's Disease, held in Noordwijk/Leiden, The Netherlands (1980). 1981 ISBN 90–247–2475–9
2. P.M. Motta and L.J.A. Didio (eds.): *Basic and Clinical Hepatology*. 1982 ISBN 90–247–2404–X
3. D. Rachmilewitz (ed.): *Inflammatory Bowel Diseases*. Proceedings of the 1st International Symposium, held in Jerusalem, Israel (1981). 1982 ISBN 90–247–2612–3
4. D. Fleischer, D. Jensen and P. Bright-Asare (eds.): *Therapeutic Laser Endoscopy in Gastrointestinal Disease*. 1983 ISBN 0–89838–577–6
5. S.P. Borriello (ed.): *Antibiotic Associated Diarrhoea and Colitis*. The Role of *Clostridium difficile* in Gastrointestinal Disorders. 1984 ISBN 0–89838–623–3
6. Ch.H. Gips and R.A.F. Krom (eds.): *Progress in Liver Transplantation*. 1985 ISBN 0–89838–726–4
7. G.F. Nelis, J. Boevé and J.J. Misiewicz (eds.): *Peptic Ulcer Disease: Basic and Clinical Aspects*. Proceedings of a Symposium on Peptic Ulcer Today, held at the Sophia Ziekenhuis, Zwolle, The Netherlands (1984). 1985 ISBN 0–89838–759–0
8. D. Rachmilewitz (ed.): *Inflammatory Bowel Diseases 1986*. Proceedings of the 2nd International Symposium, held in Jerusalem, Israel (1985). 1986 ISBN 0–89838–796–5
9. E.M.H. Mathus-Vliegen: *The Role of Laser in Gastroenterology*. Analysis of Eight Years' Experience. 1989 ISBN 0–7923–0425–X
10. D.M. Jensen and J.-M. Brunetaud (eds.): *Medical Laser Endoscopy*. 1990 ISBN 0–7923–0579–5
11. D. Rachmilewitz and J. Zimmerman (eds.): *Inflammatory Bowel Diseases 1990*. Proceedings of the 3rd International Symposium, held in Jerusalem, Israel (1989). 1990 ISBN 0–7923–0657–0
12. L. Capocaccia, G. Ricci, F. Angelico, M. Angelico, A.F. Attili and L. Lalloni (eds.): *Recent Advances in the Epidemiology and Prevention of Gallstone Disease*. Proceedings of the 2nd International Workshop, held in Rome, Italy (1989). 1991 ISBN 0-7923-0994-4
13. M.L. Mearin and C.J.J. Mulder (eds.): *Coeliac Disease*. 40 Years Gluten Free. 1991 ISBN 0-7923-1160-4
14. C.J.J. Mulder and G.N.J. Tytgat (eds.): *Is Crohn's Disease a Mycobacterial Disease ?* 1992 ISBN 0-7923-2026-3

Kluwer Academic Publishers – Dordrecht / Boston / London

MIX
Papier aus verantwortungsvollen Quellen
Paper from responsible sources
FSC® C105338

If you have any concerns about our products,
you can contact us on
ProductSafety@springernature.com

In case Publisher is established outside the EU,
the EU authorized representative is:
Springer Nature Customer Service Center GmbH
Europaplatz 3, 69115 Heidelberg, Germany

Printed by Libri Plureos GmbH
in Hamburg, Germany